THE GUT-BRAIN CONNECTION: A HOLISTIC APPROACH

DIETARY CHOICES TO REGULATE DIGESTION, BALANCE HORMONES, ENHANCE MENTAL CLARITY AND PROMOTE AUTOIMMUNE HEALTH FROM WITHIN

N.R. STERLING

© **Copyright HVNLY Publishing 2025 - All rights reserved.**

The content within this book may not be reproduced, duplicated or transmitted without direct written permission from the author or the publisher.

Under no circumstances will any blame or legal responsibility be held against the publisher, or author, for any damages, reparation, or monetary loss due to the information contained within this book. Either directly or indirectly. You are responsible for your own choices, actions, and results.

Legal Notice:

This book is copyright protected. This book is only for personal use. You cannot amend, distribute, sell, use, quote or paraphrase any part, of the content within this book, without the consent of the author or publisher.

Disclaimer Notice:

Please note the information contained within this document is for educational and entertainment purposes only. All effort has been expended to present accurate, up-to-date, and reliable, complete information. No warranties of any kind are declared or implied. Readers acknowledge that the author is not engaging in the rendering of legal, financial, medical or professional advice. The content within this book has been derived from various sources. Please consult a licensed professional before attempting any techniques outlined in this book.

By reading this document, the reader agrees that under no circumstances is the author responsible for any losses, direct or indirect, which are incurred as a result of the use of the information contained within this document, including, but not limited to, — errors, omissions, or inaccuracies.

TABLE OF CONTENTS

Introduction 7

1. UNDERSTANDING THE GUT-BRAIN AXIS 9
   The Gut-Brain Superhighway: Messages, Mood, and Balance 9
   Life Within: The Microscopic World Shaping Your Health 10
   Mood on the Menu: Serotonin's Gut Connection ... 11
   Breaking Down the Science 14
   Common Myths About the Gut-Brain Connection ... 15

2. THE IMPORTANCE OF HOLISTIC WELLNESS 17
   Addressing Misconceptions and Objections 18
   Integrating Mind-Body Practices 20
   Neuroplasticity and the Gut-Brain Connection 21
   Holistic Wellness Success Case Studies 25

3. DIET'S IMPACT ON GUT AND BRAIN 27
   The Role of Natural Prebiotics and Probiotics 27
   Prebiotics Foods 28
   Probiotic Foods 30
   Cheeses and Synbiotics 31
   The Fermented Revolution: Sauerkraut and Kimchi . 33
   Anti-Inflammatory Diet: Reducing Brain Fog and Fatigue 36
   Sugar, Gluten, and Dairy: Understanding Their Impact on Mental Clarity 37

4. HERBAL REMEDIES AND NATURAL SUPPORTS ... 41
   How Herbal Remedies Support the Gut-Brain Connection 41
   A Complete Guide to Herbs and Teas 42
   Key Herbs and their Specific Benefits 43
   Herbal Tea Recipes 46
   Customizing Recipes 51
   Essential Oils and the Gut-Brain Axis 60

Calming and Stress-Reducing Essential Oils	61
Digestive-Supporting Essential Oils	62
Mood-Enhancing and Gut-Brain Axis Oils	63
Immune-Boosting and Anti-Inflammatory Essential Oils	64
Blends and Recipes	65
Supplements for Gut-Brain Wellness	66
Incorporating Adaptogens	67
5. THE MICROBIOME'S ROLE IN MENTAL HEALTH	**69**
PTSD and Gut Bacteria: Healing Trauma from Within	69
OCD: Can Gut Health Offer New Hope?	70
Anxiety Alleviation: Probiotics as a Natural Remedy	72
Depression and the Gut: Unraveling the Connection	72
6. ADDRESSING SPECIFIC MENTAL HEALTH CONDITIONS	**75**
ADHD: Enhancing Focus through Gut Optimization	75
Dementia: The Gut's Role in Cognitive Health	76
Bipolar Disorder: Stabilizing Mood with Nutritional Interventions	78
Autism Spectrum Disorders (ASD) and the Gut-Brain Connection	78
Parkinson's Disease and Gut Health	79
7. NATURAL APPROACH FOR AUTOIMMUNE CONDITIONS	**81**
Understanding Gut Health and Inflammation	81
Food vs. Autoimmune Conditions	83
Anti-Inflammatory Foods to Include:	84
Natural Remedies for Autoimmune Symptom Relief	87
8. OTHER CONDITIONS DIRECTLY ASSOCIATED WITH GUT HEALTH	**89**
Gastrointestinal Disorders	92
Metabolic and Endocrine Disorders	93
Immune and Inflammatory Conditions	94
Cardiovascular Diseases	94
Cancer	95
Chronic Fatigue Syndrome (CFS)	96
Kidney Disease	96
Thyroid Disorders	97

Combating Insomnia: Gut Health for a Good Night's Sleep — 97
Leaky Gut and Bad Metabolites - Their Influence on Disease — 99

9. RECOGNIZING SIGNS OF GUT-RELATED ISSUES — 101
   Physical Symptoms of Gut Imbalance — 101
   Mental Symptoms of Gut Distress — 102
   When to Seek Professional Help — 103
   Who Can Help with Gut Problems? — 104
   What to Expect at Your Appointment — 104
   Treatment Options — 104
   Self-Assessment Tools for Early Detection — 105

10. DETOXIFYING GUT AND MIND — 107
    The Role of Hydration in Cleansing — 109
    Mental Detox Techniques for Clarity — 111
    Integrating Detox into a Daily Routine — 113

11. LIFESTYLE CHANGES FOR GUT-BRAIN HARMONY — 115
    Boosting Gut Health Through Movement — 115
    Tools for Emotional Balance — 117

12. MANAGING STRESS FOR GUT-BRAIN HEALTH — 119
    Understanding Stress — 119
    Cortisol's Impact on Gut Health — 121
    Stress Reduction Mindfulness Practices — 123
    Quick Stress-Reduction Techniques — 126

13. SUPPORTING THE MICROBIOME AND ADAPTING YOUR JOURNEY FOR SUSTAINABILITY — 131
    The Importance of Tracking Progress — 133
    Adjusting Dietary and Lifestyle Habits — 135
    Personalizing Your Gut-Brain Wellness Plan — 136
    Maintaining Motivation and Overcoming Setbacks — 138
    Cultivating a Growth Mindset for Personal Development — 139

    RECIPES : SEVEN-DAY MEAL PLAN — 141
    Breakfast Recipes — 141
    Lunch Recipes — 145
    Dinner Recipes — 149

Snack Recipes	152
Optional Add-Ons	155
Making Fermented Carrots	160
Making Sauerkraut	163
Making Kimchi	165
Tempeh and its Key Features	167
Health Benefits of Tempeh	168
Tempeh vs. Tofu	168
Making Tempeh	169
How to Use Homemade Tempeh:	172
Conclusion	175
References	181

INTRODUCTION

We often hear that the gut is our second brain. But what if I told you it might be more like our first? Recent studies reveal that the gut and brain communicate constantly, influencing everything from mood swings to anxiety levels. A healthy gut can lead to a healthy mind, a connection that's now at the forefront of medical science. Understanding it can transform not just how we eat but how we live.

In this book, we'll explore how the physical, mental, and emotional aspects of our well-being are intertwined. A holistic approach isn't just about food or exercise. It's about seeing ourselves as whole beings, where every part affects the other. By focusing on the gut-brain connection, we can address multiple aspects of our health at once.

So, if you are a health enthusiast, someone dealing with stress-related digestive issues, or just curious about preventative health, this book is definitely for you. And whatever your background, this book offers unique insights into how you can improve your well-being.

From nourishing your gut with the right foods to managing stress effectively, you'll learn all about prebiotics and probiotics and how they can transform your digestive health. We'll also look into how to recognize the signs of gut-related issues and understand their impact on mental clarity and emotional balance.

My interest in the gut-brain connection began years ago when I noticed how stress impacted both my digestion and mood. Since then, I've spent years researching, attending seminars, and meeting with experts to learn more.

The book is written sequentially so that it can guide you step-by-step. You'll start by understanding the gut-brain axis and why holistic wellness matters. Then, you'll discover how to nourish your gut and recognize signs of imbalance. Later, you'll learn about the role your gut plays in both your mental and emotional health and how managing stress can improve your health.

As you read, you'll find actionable steps and strategies to enhance your gut-brain health. This is a practical guide designed to bring real change. You'll learn how to create a gut-friendly meal plan, incorporate stress-reduction techniques, and track your progress. These tools will empower you to take control of your health journey.

UNDERSTANDING THE GUT-BRAIN AXIS

Through the gut-brain axis, your physical, mental, and emotional health are connected. It's not just about what you eat; it's about how you live. Mood regulation, immune system modulation, and stress management all find their roots in this axis. A holistic health perspective combines these elements, emphasizing the importance of a balanced lifestyle. It invites you to consider not just diet but also stress management and mind-body therapies as integral parts of maintaining a healthy gut-brain relationship.

THE GUT-BRAIN SUPERHIGHWAY: MESSAGES, MOOD, AND BALANCE

Imagine a busy highway where information travels at lightning speed from one part of the body to another. This is much like the vagus nerve, an important player in our body's communication system, which stretches from the gut to the brain. It carries information, ensuring that the two organs are in constant communication. But it doesn't do this on its own. Peptides like ghrelin and leptin also play a part, relaying signals about hunger and satiety.

Like little messengers, they keep the brain up to date on the body's needs.

Beyond these pathways, hormones and neurotransmitters act as mediators in this relationship. Cortisol, often called the stress hormone, can wreak havoc on gut function during times of stress. Serotonin, on the other hand, is a mood regulator produced both in the brain and the gut. It impacts how we feel emotionally and affects our gut's function. Then there's dopamine, a neurotransmitter involved in gut-brain signaling, which plays a part in how we experience pleasure and satisfaction. These chemicals balance our mood, digestion, and overall health.

The immune system also plays a part, with gut-associated lymphoid tissue (GALT) monitoring and responding to potential threats. It communicates with the brain through inflammation pathways and cytokine signaling. This relationship between the gut, brain, and immune system maintains harmony within the body.

*Reflect on a stressful day when you noticed changes in your digestion or mood. Jot down any patterns or triggers you observed. Consider how understanding these communication pathways might help you manage those symptoms in the future.

LIFE WITHIN: THE MICROSCOPIC WORLD SHAPING YOUR HEALTH

Inside your gut, trillions of microorganisms, including bacteria, viruses, fungi, and archaea form the microbiome, which outnumbers the amount of human cells in your body. Each microbe plays a vital role in maintaining balance. When the balance tips, health issues can arise. A varied microbiome supports digestion, immunity, and even mood regulation. Each microbe contributes to breaking down complex carbohydrates into simpler forms that your body can use for energy. They synthesize essential vitamins, like B and K, that your body can't produce on its own, and they stand guard against pathogens, effectively keeping you healthy.

The balance of this ecosystem is very delicate, influenced by what you eat, where you live, and even the medications you take. Antibiotics, while life-saving, can disrupt this balance, wiping out both harmful and beneficial bacteria. A diet rich in fiber and fermented foods can nurture your microbiome, feeding good bacteria and promoting their growth. Meanwhile, pollution and other environmental factors can alter the microbiome's composition, sometimes leading to dysbiosis. Dysbiosis is imbalance in the microbiome, which can lead to everything from obesity and diabetes to mental health disorders.

Today, there's a growing interest in therapies that leverage the gut-brain connection to restore balance. Fecal microbiota transplantation (FMT), for example, involves transferring stool from a healthy donor to a patient and has shown promise in treating certain infections and gut-related diseases. Personalized nutrition plans, tailored to an individual's microbiome, are also a popular way to optimize health. These therapies aim to rebalance the microbiome by providing a custom approach that considers your unique microbial landscape.

MOOD ON THE MENU: SEROTONIN'S GUT CONNECTION

In regards to our gut and mood, neurotransmitters play a starring role. Among them, serotonin, often dubbed the "feel-good" chemical, is a major player. Surprisingly, a significant portion of serotonin is actually produced in the gut, not the brain. This production site makes the gut a central hub for mood regulation. When our serotonin levels are balanced, we tend to feel more emotionally stable. However, when they're out of sync, mood disorders such as depression and anxiety can develop.

The path serotonin travels begins with tryptophan, an amino acid found in various foods. Once ingested, tryptophan transforms into serotonin. This conversion is why it's important to follow a diet rich in tryptophan, found in foods like turkey, nuts, and seeds. Once synthesized, serotonin is released into the bloodstream, eventually making its way to the brain where it influences mood and behavior. The interaction between serotonin and its receptors is crucial in determining how effectively the neurotransmitter can exert its calming effects on the mind.

High-Tryptophan Foods

Animal-Based Sources

1. **Turkey**
    - A well-known source, often linked to its sleep-inducing effects.
    - Serving: 100g provides ~350mg of tryptophan.
2. **Chicken**
    - High in tryptophan, especially in the breast meat.
    - Serving: 100g provides ~300mg.
3. **Eggs**
    - Particularly the yolk, which is rich in tryptophan.
    - Serving: One large egg provides ~70mg.
4. **Fish**
    - Examples: Salmon, cod, tuna, and halibut are excellent sources.
    - Serving: 100g provides ~250–300mg.

5. **Dairy Products**
   - Examples: Milk, cheese (e.g., cheddar, Parmesan), and yogurt.
   - Serving: One cup of milk provides ~100mg; cheese varies by type.
6. **Beef and Lamb**
   - Red meats are moderate sources of tryptophan.
   - Serving: 100g provides ~250mg.
7. **Pork**
   - Rich in tryptophan, especially in lean cuts.
   - Serving: 100g provides ~250–300mg.

Plant-Based Sources

1. **Nuts and Seeds**
   - Examples: Almonds, walnuts, sunflower seeds, pumpkin seeds, sesame seeds.
   - Serving: 1 ounce of pumpkin seeds provides ~100mg of tryptophan.
2. **Soy Products**
   - Examples: Tofu, tempeh, soy milk, and edamame.
   - Serving: 100g of tofu provides ~120mg.
3. **Legumes**
   - Examples: Lentils, chickpeas, black beans, kidney beans.
   - Serving: 1 cup of lentils provides ~180mg.
4. **Whole Grains**
   - Examples: Oats, quinoa, barley, and brown rice.
   - Serving: 1 cup of cooked oats provides ~50mg.
5. **Fruits**
   - Examples: Bananas, pineapples, and kiwis.
   - Serving: One banana provides ~10mg.

6. **Vegetables**
   - Examples: Spinach, kale, broccoli, and asparagus.
   - Serving: 1 cup of cooked spinach provides ~40mg.
7. **Dark Chocolate**
   - Contains tryptophan as well as mood-enhancing polyphenols.
   - Serving: 1 ounce provides ~30mg.

Tips to Maximize Tryptophan Absorption

- **Combine with Carbohydrates:** Carbs stimulate insulin, which helps transport tryptophan to the brain. Pair tryptophan-rich foods with whole grains, fruits, or starchy vegetables.
  - Example: Turkey with quinoa or banana with yogurt.
- **Include B Vitamins and Magnesium:** These nutrients help convert tryptophan into serotonin.
  - **Sources:** Leafy greens, nuts, seeds, and fortified cereals.

Lifestyle choices also play an important role in serotonin production. Stress, for instance, can deplete serotonin levels. Similarly, inadequate sleep can throw off the body's natural rhythm, reducing serotonin availability. Maintaining gut health is vital for optimal serotonin synthesis. Eating a balanced diet, managing stress effectively, and prioritizing restful sleep are all ways you can support neurotransmitter production. Effectively, our choices shape our mental makeup, with serotonin acting as a bridge between our physical and emotional health.

BREAKING DOWN THE SCIENCE

The conversation between your gut and brain occurs on a **molecular** level. Imagine neural pathways as roads bustling with signals, where synaptic transmissions serve as the vehicles carrying messages between neurons. These pathways ensure that the gut and brain remain connected, exchanging information about everything from hunger to fear. Hormonal signaling adds another layer to this complex network. Hormones act like messengers, relaying information that can influence mood, digestion, and even decision-making.

The gut microbiota produces short-chain fatty acids, which influence brain function and behavior. These acids can cross the blood-brain barrier, impacting cognition and mood. These microbes modulate the immune system, ensuring it remains vigilant yet not overactive. This modulation is important, as an overactive immune response can lead to inflammation, affecting both gut and brain health.

Emerging research and technologies continue to shed light on this communication. Fecal transplants, once an unorthodox treatment, are now believed to restore microbial balance, helping conditions like depression or anxiety. Neuroimaging techniques, meanwhile, provide a window into the brain's response to gut stimuli, allowing researchers to observe real-time changes in brain activity in response to gut-derived signals.

The potential applications of this research are vast and could transform treatment options, moving away from one-size-fits-all solutions to more personalized and effective strategies.

COMMON MYTHS ABOUT THE GUT-BRAIN CONNECTION

There's a common misconception that our gut is just a digestive organ, tirelessly processing food and doing nothing more. But this couldn't be further from the truth. As previously discussed, the gut is a sophisticated system linked to our mood, health, and overall well-being. When we dismiss the gut as merely a food processor, we ignore its profound impact on our mental and emotional states.

Another misconception is that only extreme diets can impact gut health. Really, small, consistent dietary changes can make a huge difference. You don't have to overhaul your entire diet overnight. Instead, integrate more fiber-rich foods, fermented products, and a variety of nutrients that can gradually nurture your gut. The idea that drastic measures are often required leads to unnecessary stress and unsustainable habits.

The difference between probiotics and prebiotics is another area of confusion. Probiotics are live bacteria found in foods or supplements that are beneficial for gut health. Prebiotics, on the other hand, are types of fiber that feed these good bacteria. Understanding this distinction helps us make better choices about what our bodies need.

There's also a damaging myth that gut health can't affect severe mental health conditions. This underestimates the gut's role in emotional regulation and mental health. Research shows that gut imbalances can influence conditions like anxiety and depression. By caring for our gut, we can indirectly support our mental health.

Embracing information means recognizing the value of personalized health strategies. Each of us is unique, and our health needs are no exception. What's beneficial for one person may not work for another. Staying educated and adaptable allows us to navigate health information and take proactive steps toward better health.

THE IMPORTANCE OF HOLISTIC WELLNESS

Holistic wellness goes beyond conventional health practices by addressing the entire person rather than isolated symptoms. By focusing on the interconnectedness of body, mind, and spirit, holistic wellness offers a path to complete and sustainable health.

Adopting a holistic approach to health offers many benefits. For instance, a balanced lifestyle enhances immune function, making you more resilient to everyday illnesses. By nurturing your entire self, you build a foundation of well-being that supports everything from your immune system to your emotional resilience.

One of the strengths of holistic practices lies in long-term sustainability. Unlike quick fixes that often rely on medication, holistic wellness encourages us to create lifelong healthy habits. Habits that reduce the need for chronic medication by addressing causes rather than just symptoms. The beauty of this approach is its adaptability, allowing you to tailor practices to suit your lifestyle and personal needs, ensuring they remain a permanent part of your daily routine.

Holistic wellness also brings emotional and psychological benefits. By focusing on the whole person, you cultivate practices like mindfulness and balanced nutrition that enhance your mental health and help you maintain equilibrium. You become more in tune with your emotions and able to process and respond to them effectively.

Additionally, community and social support play a big role in holistic health. Building a supportive network and engaging in group activities, such as yoga classes or meditation, fosters a sense of belonging.

Reflection:

Consider the areas of your life where you could include more holistic practices. What small changes can you make in your daily routine to support your physical, mental, and emotional well-being? Reflect on the role of community in your wellness journey and how you might engage with others to foster a supportive environment.

ADDRESSING MISCONCEPTIONS AND OBJECTIONS

Holistic health often gets a bad rap for being unscientific and is dismissed by skeptics as a pseudoscience. Yet, this overlooks the growing body of research supporting holistic practices. For instance, psychoneuroimmunology studies how our mental states can influence immune function, revealing the scientific basis behind mind-body connections. Critics may argue that holistic methods lack rigorous testing, but they ignore their ability to integrate ancient wisdom with modern science. Holistic health encompasses all lifestyle aspects of human well-being. The science is there, just waiting to be embraced.

Some people think adopting a holistic lifestyle is too time-consuming, requiring hours of yoga or meditation daily. But that's simply not true. Even small changes can make a big difference. Integrating mindfulness into your daily routine can be as simple as taking a few minutes to breathe deeply during breaks. It's about making thoughtful choices, like choosing whole foods over processed ones or taking a short walk after dinner. These practices fit into any schedule and are all about finding what works for you without upending your life.

Cost is another big concern. Many believe holistic health is expensive, reserved for those with disposable income to spend on organic foods or wellness retreats. However, plenty of low-cost or free resources are available, from online yoga classes to community gardens offering fresh produce. Swapping out costly supplements for nutrient-rich foods can also save money while providing more significant health benefits. The key is to prioritize what you can change within your budget.

Skepticism is fueled by a culture that favors quick fixes. Many people want immediate results from a pill or a fad diet, overlooking the importance of gradual lifestyle changes. Holistic health encourages a shift in mindset, focusing on sustainable practices that nurture long-term health. Quick solutions are appealing, but they rarely address underlying issues. Taking the time to build healthy habits definitely pays off in the long run.

More and more healthcare professionals are endorsing holistic approaches. Dr. Andrew Weil, a pioneer in integrative medicine, advocates for combining conventional and holistic practices to improve health outcomes. He emphasizes the importance of balance, suggesting that holistic methods complement traditional treatments rather than replace them.

INTEGRATING MIND-BODY PRACTICES

Too often, the connection between mind and body takes a backseat. Yet, this connection can profoundly transform our health, especially when focusing on gut-brain wellness. Mind-body practices like yoga and meditation play an important role here. Yoga, an ancient practice, is renowned for its ability to reduce inflammation. By engaging in gentle movements and focused breathing, yoga stimulates the parasympathetic nervous system, also known as the rest-and-digest system. This activation helps lower cortisol levels, the stress hormone that can majorly impact your body and mind. Yoga also helps establish a sense of tranquility and clarity, aiding in stress reduction and mental focus. Meditation, on the other hand, has been shown to improve mental clarity. Regular meditation can rewire your brain, reduce stress, and help you cope with challenges.

Incorporating these practices into your routine doesn't require drastic changes. Start small. Consider beginning your day with a brief meditation session, even if it's just five minutes. This can reset your mind and ease tension, creating a ripple effect throughout your day. Gradually, you might extend your practice, exploring different styles of yoga or meditation to find what works best for you. The goal is to integrate these practices into your life.

The scientific foundation of mind-body practices is compelling. Yoga and meditation can lower cortisol levels, not only improving your mental health but also positively impacting gut health. When stress decreases, the gut functions more efficiently, improving digestion and supporting a diverse microbiome. A balanced microbiome is necessary for overall health, as it plays a major role in processing nutrients and supporting immune function. By reducing stress, you allow beneficial bacteria to thrive, enhancing your gut-brain connection.

These practices extend beyond just physical well-being. They offer a holistic approach to health that recognizes the interconnectedness of body and mind.

NEUROPLASTICITY AND THE GUT-BRAIN CONNECTION

Neuroplasticity refers to the brain's remarkable ability to reorganize itself by forming new neural connections. This adaptability allows the brain to recover from injuries, adapt to new situations, and even change in response to learning. The gut-brain axis plays a significant role in this process. Our gut health can actually influence how effectively our brain adapts and reorganizes. The microbiome, that community of microorganisms in our gut, helps your brain stay healthy by creating special chemicals (called metabolites) that encourage the growth of new brain cells, a process known as neurogenesis. These chemicals also keep the connections between brain cells flexible and strong, which is important for learning, memory, and adapting to new experiences. This flexibility, called synaptic plasticity, helps your brain work better and can even make you more emotionally resilient.

Diet is a powerful tool in shaping neuroplasticity, with certain diets showing a positive impact on brain health. Surely you've heard the saying " You are what you eat"? Well, it's true. The Mediterranean diet, rich in fruits, vegetables, whole grains, and healthy fats, is particularly beneficial. It supports neuroplasticity by providing the brain with essential nutrients and antioxidants that promote cell health and repair. Foods like olive oil, nuts, and fatty fish are excellent sources of omega-3 fatty acids, which are known for their role in brain function and development. These nutrients support the structural integrity of brain cells and enhance communication between neurons. By nourishing the gut with these wholesome foods, we indirectly support our brain's ability to adapt and thrive.

Mediterranean Diet

The Mediterranean diet emphasizes whole, minimally processed foods, mindful eating, and active living. It's flexible, making it easy to adapt to personal preferences and dietary needs.

Key Components

1. **Plant-Based Focus**
   - Emphasis on vegetables, fruits, whole grains, nuts, seeds, and legumes.
   - These are rich in fiber, vitamins, minerals, and antioxidants.
2. **Healthy Fats**
   - Primary source: **extra-virgin olive oil** (used for cooking, dressings, and more).
   - Other sources: nuts, seeds, and fatty fish (rich in omega-3 fatty acids).
3. **Moderate Protein Intake**
   - **Fish and seafood**: Consumed at least twice a week. Includes salmon, sardines, mackerel, and tuna.
   - **Poultry and eggs**: Eaten in moderation.
   - **Dairy**: Focus on low-fat or moderate amounts of yogurt and cheese.
4. **Limited Red Meat**
   - Red meat is eaten sparingly, usually in small portions or as part of a dish.

5. **Minimized Processed Foods and Sugars**
   - Avoidance of heavily processed foods, added sugars, and refined grains.
6. **Herbs and Spices**
   - Flavor dishes with fresh herbs, garlic, and spices instead of salt.
7. **Wine (Optional)**
   - Moderate consumption of red wine (up to one glass per day for women and two for men), if it aligns with personal and cultural preferences.

Daily Guidelines

- **Vegetables**: Aim for a variety (e.g., leafy greens, tomatoes, peppers, zucchini). At least 2 servings per meal.
- **Fruits**: 2–3 servings daily as snacks or desserts.
- **Whole Grains**: Include options like whole-grain bread, brown rice, quinoa, and barley.
- **Nuts and Seeds**: A small handful daily as snacks or toppings.
- **Legumes**: Include beans, lentils, and chickpeas several times a week.

Weekly Guidelines

- **Fish and Seafood**: 2–3 servings.
- **Poultry and Eggs**: Moderate amounts, such as 1–2 servings.
- **Dairy**: Enjoy low-fat yogurt or cheese in moderation.

Occasional Treats

- **Red Meat**: A few times per month in small portions.
- **Sweets**: Rarely, and when consumed, opt for natural sweeteners like honey.

Lifestyle Aspects

1. **Social Eating**: Share meals with family and friends to enhance satisfaction and mindfulness.
2. **Physical Activity**: Regular exercise is a key part of the Mediterranean lifestyle.
3. **Mindfulness**: Slow down and savor your meals.

Health Benefits

- **Heart Health**: Reduces the risk of cardiovascular disease.
- **Brain Health**: Associated with improved cognitive function and reduced risk of Alzheimer's.
- **Weight Management**: Encourages nutrient-dense, satisfying meals.
- **Inflammation**: Helps lower inflammation in the body.
- **Longevity**: Linked to a longer, healthier life.

Integrating cognitive enhancement practices can also help brain adaptability. Simple brain exercises, such as puzzles and memory games, can stimulate neuroplasticity. When you add a gut-friendly diet, these activities become even more effective. Mindful meditation is another powerful practice that enhances gut-brain communication. As you incorporate these practices into your daily routine, you'll notice improvements in memory, focus, and even emotional balance.

The interplay between neuroplasticity and gut health is a testament to the body's incredible ability to heal and adapt. By understanding this connection, you open the door to enhanced cognitive functions and a more resilient mind. Follow a balanced diet, engage in regular mental exercises, and practice mindfulness to transform the way your brain and gut interact, leading to improved mental clarity and overall well-being.

HOLISTIC WELLNESS SUCCESS CASE STUDIES

Ana, a good friend of mine of many years, is a middle-aged professional who struggled with irritable bowel syndrome (IBS) for years. Her symptoms were relentless, affecting every aspect of her life. Frustrated by conventional treatments, she turned to a holistic approach and incorporated dietary changes, regular exercise, and mindfulness techniques. She eliminated certain trigger foods and followed a diet rich in whole grains, fruits, and probiotics. She also practiced mindfulness, which helped manage her stress levels. Over time, her IBS symptoms lessened, and she found herself using fewer medications.

John, a high-school teacher in his 50's, was dealing with chronic stress and fatigue. His job left him feeling drained and overwhelmed. He incorporated a blend of holistic strategies, including a balanced diet, tai chi, and deep breathing exercises to help him better manage his stress. He says that within a few months, he experienced a noticeable boost in energy and mental clarity, which allowed him to engage more actively with his students and family.

Many individuals report quantifiable improvements, such as reduced reliance on medications and improved health metrics. For instance, a study of holistic practices found that participants reported a 30% reduction in medication use after adopting a holistic health regimen, alongside enhanced emotional resilience and improved sleep patterns. Another study published in the *North American Spine Society Journal* found that a 12-week program combining qigong and t'ai chi significantly improved back pain, physical function, and sleep quality in participants.

Across different ages and lifestyles, people have embraced these practices, overcoming cultural barriers and personal challenges. As we move forward, we'll explore more strategies to deepen our understanding of the gut-brain connection and how it influences our wellness.

DIET'S IMPACT ON GUT AND BRAIN

In a previous chapter, we compared the gut to a busy city where trillions of microscopic citizens work tirelessly to support our well-being. But just like anything else, they need the right resources to flourish. This is where prebiotics and probiotics come in.

THE ROLE OF NATURAL PREBIOTICS AND PROBIOTICS

Prebiotics provide the nutrients that beneficial bacteria need to thrive. These are non-digestible fibers found in foods like garlic, onions, chicory root and asparagus that pass through your digestive system mostly undigested. Prebiotics feed your gut's good bacteria, promoting their growth and activity, and supporting functions like digestion and immune response.

PREBIOTICS FOODS

Vegetables

1. Garlic
2. Onions
3. Leeks
4. Asparagus
5. Jerusalem artichokes (sunchokes)
6. Dandelion greens
7. Chicory root
8. Cauliflower
9. Broccoli
10. Brussels sprouts

Fruits

1. Bananas (especially slightly green ones)
2. Apples (with the skin)
3. Berries (e.g., blueberries, raspberries, strawberries)
4. Pomegranates
5. Watermelon

Grains and Legumes

1. Oats (whole or steel-cut)
2. Barley
3. Whole wheat
4. Rye
5. Chickpeas
6. Lentils
7. Black beans
8. Kidney beans

Nuts and Seeds

1. Flaxseeds
2. Chia seeds
3. Almonds
4. Pistachios

Other Foods

1. Cocoa (unsweetened or dark chocolate with high cocoa content)
2. Seaweed (e.g., nori, wakame, kombu)
3. Potatoes (cooked and cooled, as they contain resistant starch)
4. Rice (cooked and cooled, for resistant starch)

Probiotics, on the other hand, are live bacteria that boost the population of beneficial microbes in your gut. These are found in fermented foods like yogurt and kefir, rich in live cultures. Probiotics help the existing bacteria in your gut and aid digestion and nutrient absorption. They prevent the growth of harmful bacteria, improving digestion, and influencing mental well-being.

Probiotics can also be taken as supplements, which are convenient for those who may not consume enough fermented foods regularly. When selecting probiotic supplements, try to choose products containing diverse strains that are stored properly to ensure freshness. Opt for brands that have undergone rigorous testing to guarantee their effectiveness.

PROBIOTIC FOODS

Dairy-Based Probiotic Foods

1. Yogurt (with live active cultures)
2. Kefir (fermented milk drink)
3. Buttermilk (traditional, not cultured)
4. Cheese (aged varieties with live cultures like gouda, cheddar, and Parmesan)

Fermented Vegetables

1. Sauerkraut (unpasteurized)
2. Kimchi
3. Pickles (fermented, not vinegar-brined)
4. Fermented carrots
5. Fermented beets

Soy-Based Probiotic Foods

1. Miso (fermented soybean paste)
2. Tempeh (fermented soybean cake)
3. Natto (fermented soybeans)

Grain-Based Probiotic Foods

1. Sourdough bread (made with natural fermentation)
2. Idli (fermented rice and lentil cakes)
3. Dosa (fermented rice and lentil crepes)

Fermented Drinks

1. Kombucha (fermented tea)
2. Kvass (fermented rye drink)
3. Jun tea (similar to kombucha, made with green tea and honey)
4. Yakult (fermented milk drink)

Other Probiotic Foods

1. Fermented garlic
2. Fermented chili paste (e.g., gochujang)
3. Umeboshi (fermented Japanese plums)
4. Fermented fish (e.g., fish sauce, pla ra, surströmming)

When prebiotics and probiotics are consumed together, they create an effect called synbiotics, which enhance gut health even more effectively than either could alone. By providing both the bacteria (probiotics) and their food (prebiotics), you can increase the diversity of the gut microbiota, which is crucial for the digestive system.

Synbiotics can be found in certain foods, such as cheese and kefir, where both prebiotics and probiotics coexist.

CHEESES AND SYNBIOTICS

Not all types of cheese contain synbiotics.

What are Synbiotics?

Synbiotics are a combination of probiotics (beneficial bacteria) and prebiotics (food for those bacteria) that work together to support gut health.

1. **Probiotics in Cheese**:
   - Many fermented cheeses, such as certain types of cheddar, gouda, blue cheese, and Parmesan, may contain probiotics, especially if they are unpasteurized or specially cultured with live bacteria.
   - Probiotics may survive the cheese-making process, depending on the strain used, aging, and storage conditions.
2. **Prebiotics in Cheese**:
   - Some cheeses contain prebiotic components, like certain fibers or oligosaccharides, but not all.
   - Additional prebiotics may sometimes be added during processing to enhance health benefits.
3. **Synbiotic Potential**:
   - Cheeses that naturally retain live bacteria and also have prebiotic components (like inulin-enriched or fiber-enhanced cheeses) can be considered synbiotics.
   - A common example is aged gouda, which contains live bacteria and galactooligosaccharides, a natural prebiotic.

Cheeses Without Synbiotics

- Processed cheeses, pasteurized cheeses, and cheeses with no live bacterial cultures that typically lack probiotics.
- Hard or aged cheeses that undergo processes eliminating live bacteria may also not qualify.

To confirm if a specific cheese has synbiotic properties, check the packaging.

Incorporating prebiotics and probiotics into your routine can be simple and delicious. Start your day with a yogurt parfait topped with sliced bananas and a sprinkle of oats for a combination of probiotics and prebiotics. Then, sip on a refreshing glass of kefir as a midday snack and later add some garlic and asparagus to your evening stir-fry for a gut-friendly meal. Experiment with ingredients to find your favorite combinations and note any changes in your digestion or mood over time.

THE FERMENTED REVOLUTION: SAUERKRAUT AND KIMCHI

Fermentation is a natural process through which microorganisms like bacteria, yeast, and molds convert sugars and starch into alcohol or acids. This process doesn't just preserve food; it enhances its nutritional value and makes it easier for our bodies to absorb vital nutrients.

Fermented foods introduce beneficial bacteria that diversify the gut microbiome. A diverse gut flora helps maintain a balanced digestive system and supports overall health. These foods can help reduce inflammation, a common culprit behind many chronic diseases and mental health issues. By reducing inflammation, you can improve your mental clarity and mood. A happy gut means a happier mind with reduced symptoms of stress and fatigue.

Sauerkraut and kimchi are the two most popular fermented foods, each offering unique health benefits. Sauerkraut, made from fermented cabbage, is rich in vitamins C and K, as well as fiber and iron. Kimchi, a staple in Korean cuisine, combines fermented cabbage with a variety of spices, garlic, and ginger. Other fermented dairy products like kefir provide additional benefits. Kefir, for instance, is loaded with calcium, protein, and B vitamins, offering a creamy and tangy alternative to traditional dairy.

Incorporating fermented foods into your diet is simple and enjoyable. Start by adding a small serving of sauerkraut or kimchi as a side dish to your meals. Just a few spoonfuls can introduce an array of probiotics to your system. Homemade fermentation is also growing in popularity. If you're interested, start with basic recipes, like fermenting cabbage to make your own sauerkraut. As you become more comfortable with the process, you can experiment with different vegetables and spices to create unique flavors.

Fermented Foods:

Dairy-Based Fermented Foods

1. Yogurt (with live cultures)
2. Buttermilk (cultured)
3. Crème fraîche
4. Skyr (Icelandic cultured dairy)
5. Paneer (fermented) (in some regions)

Vegetable-Based Fermented Foods

1. Pickles (fermented, not vinegar-based)
2. Fermented carrots
3. Beet kvass
4. Fermented garlic
5. Fermented radishes

Grain-Based Fermented Foods

1. Sourdough bread
2. Idli (fermented rice and lentil cakes from India)
3. Dosa (fermented rice and lentil crepe)
4. Injera (Ethiopian fermented flatbread)
5. Rejuvelac (fermented grain drink)

Legume-Based Fermented Foods

1. Natto (fermented soybeans from Japan)
2. Tempeh (fermented soy cake from Indonesia)
3. Miso (fermented soybean paste from Japan)
4. Soy sauce (naturally brewed)
5. Fermented black beans (Chinese cuisine)

Beverages

1. Kombucha (fermented tea)
2. Kvass (fermented rye drink)
3. Jun tea (similar to kombucha, made with green tea and honey)
4. Chicha (fermented corn drink from South America)
5. Tepache (fermented pineapple drink from Mexico)

Fish-Based Fermented Foods

1. Fish sauce (Southeast Asia)
2. Shrimp paste (fermented shrimp from Southeast Asia)
3. Hákarl (fermented shark from Iceland)
4. Pla ra (fermented fish from Thailand)
5. Surströmming (fermented herring from Sweden)

Other Fermented Foods

1. Cheese (varieties with live cultures, e.g., blue cheese, gouda)
2. Fermented honey (mead) (traditional honey fermentation)
3. Fermented mustard greens (used in Asian cuisines)
4. Fermented chili paste (e.g., sambal or gochujang)
5. Fermented plums (umeboshi) (Japanese cuisine)

Fermented foods cater to all culinary preferences. Whether you're a vegetarian, vegan, or omnivore, there are plenty of options to explore. The key is to find what you enjoy and what fits into your lifestyle.

ANTI-INFLAMMATORY DIET: REDUCING BRAIN FOG AND FATIGUE

Inflammation is the body's natural response to injury or infection, signaling your immune system to heal damaged tissue. But what happens when this alarm system gets stuck in the "on" position? Chronic inflammation can wreak havoc, particularly on the gut-brain axis. It leads to cognitive issues and even contributes to chronic diseases like heart disease and diabetes. Inflammation can lead to symptoms like brain fog, fatigue, and mood swings, making everyday tasks feel like uphill battles.

An anti-inflammatory diet works to restore balance. Omega-3 fatty acids, found in fish like salmon and plant sources like flaxseeds, help reduce inflammatory markers in the body, promoting heart health and improving cognitive function. Antioxidant-rich fruits and vegetables, such as berries, spinach, and kale, also combat oxidative stress, a significant contributor to inflammation, by neutralizing free radicals that damage cells.

Reducing inflammation through diet can lead to improved mental clarity and energy levels. When inflammation subsides, the brain can function more efficiently, enhancing both mood and focus, making it easier to concentrate and feel energized throughout the day. This allows for better decision-making, improved memory, and an overall uplift in mood.

Implementing an anti-inflammatory diet doesn't require a complete overhaul of your current eating habits. Again, start small by planning meals that include anti-inflammatory foods. For breakfast, enjoy a smoothie packed with spinach, berries, and flaxseed. Lunch could be a salad topped with grilled salmon and a variety of colorful vegetables. For dinner, consider a stir-fry with turmeric-spiced chicken and an array of greens. Turmeric, with its active compound curcumin, is renowned for its anti-inflammatory properties.

Also, remember to be mindful of what you drink. Green tea, rich in antioxidants, complements an anti-inflammatory diet well. Try swapping out sugary beverages for a cup of green tea, which can help reduce inflammation while offering a gentle energy boost. Even small changes have a significant impact.

SUGAR, GLUTEN, AND DAIRY: UNDERSTANDING THEIR IMPACT ON MENTAL CLARITY

Consuming high amounts of sugar can lead to mood swings, sending you on an emotional rollercoaster with peaks of energy followed by steep crashes. These fluctuations aren't just tiring; they can cloud your thinking, making it hard to concentrate. This cycle can disrupt your day and impact your productivity, leaving you feeling mentally foggy and drained. Therefore, limiting your sugar intake can help stabilize energy levels and mood, allowing your mind to function more smoothly and efficiently.

Gluten, a protein found in wheat and other grains, can also lead to brain fog, especially if you are sensitive to it. Dairy, too, can have cognitive effects, especially in those with lactose intolerance or a dairy allergy. Consuming dairy may lead to headaches, fatigue, or even mental confusion. Because the brain and gut are closely linked, it's no surprise that what affects one can impact the other. Understanding how these foods affect you personally is key to maintaining mental sharpness.

Elimination diets are a good way to identify food sensitivities that might be clouding your mind. By removing potential trigger foods like sugar, gluten, and dairy from your diet, you can observe changes in mental clarity and overall well-being. Begin by cutting out these foods completely, and after a few weeks, gradually reintroducing them one at a time, monitoring your body's responses closely. This reintroduction phase helps pinpoint which foods, if any, are causing problems. Keep a detailed journal during this period, noting any changes in mood, energy, or cognitive function.

For those who tolerate them, moderation is key when it comes to sugar, gluten, and dairy. Reducing sugar can start with simple swaps, like choosing whole fruits over sugary snacks or opting for water instead of soda. Reading labels can also help you spot hidden sugars in processed foods. When it comes to gluten, try gluten-free alternatives like quinoa or rice. For dairy alternatives, try almond milk, coconut yogurt, and cashew cheese. Balancing indulgence with mindfulness ensures that you enjoy these foods without overloading your system.

In the end, understanding the impact of sugar, gluten, and dairy on your mental clarity is about tuning into your body's signals and making informed choices. By finding out how these dietary components affect you personally, you can optimize your diet for better focus and energy. As we move into the next chapter, we'll explore how these insights can further enhance your overall wellness.

HERBAL REMEDIES AND NATURAL SUPPORTS

The key to balancing your gut and mind might be right in your garden or spice rack. What once seemed like an old-fashioned remedy is now backed by modern science: herbs can calm your nerves and ease your mind. They are becoming an important part of the growing focus on gut-brain health. Whether you want to reduce stress, lower inflammation, or feel better overall, herbs provide a simple way to support your health.

HOW HERBAL REMEDIES SUPPORT THE GUT-BRAIN CONNECTION

Herbs are amazing because they improve how your brain and gut work together by supporting the natural chemicals that send messages between them. For example, rosemary contains a special ingredient called *rosmarinic acid*, which can lower inflammation caused by an imbalanced gut and even help with mood problems like depression. Herbs also help balance the chemicals in your brain, which can improve your mood, reduce anxiety, and help you relax, creating a sense of calm and balance in your body.

Herbs like turmeric and boswellia are especially powerful when it comes to reducing inflammation. Turmeric contains curcumin, which calms the inflammation that can upset the balance between your gut and brain. *Curcumin* targets the causes of inflammation and is particularly helpful for conditions like irritable bowel syndrome (IBS), where inflammation is a big problem. Boswellia, another herb often used in traditional medicine, can also ease gut inflammation.

Herbs also possess calming effects on the nervous system. Valerian root helps reduce anxiety and promote restful sleep. Passionflower plays a role in promoting relaxation and emotional balance. These herbs provide a natural way to support mental clarity, nurturing a calm mind and balanced emotions.

Scientific studies support how well these herbal remedies work. Clinical trials show they can help manage symptoms of irritable bowel syndrome (IBS), a condition often made worse by stress. For example, research has found that peppermint oil can calm the gut, easing discomfort and improving digestion. These findings prove that using herbs, alongside traditional treatments, improves gut-brain health care.

A COMPLETE GUIDE TO HERBS AND TEAS

There's something undeniably comforting about a warm cup of herbal tea. However, many teas provide more than just a little comfort. Chamomile, for instance, offers gentle relief for digestive discomfort and helps enhance sleep quality. Then there's ginger, a powerhouse known for its digestive soothing and anti-inflammatory properties. Whether you're battling nausea or just want to keep your digestive system in check, ginger can help. Fennel eases bloating and gas, acting like a natural deflator, helping your body find its rhythm again.

KEY HERBS AND THEIR SPECIFIC BENEFITS

Digestive Support Herbs

These herbs improve digestion, enhance nutrient absorption, and support microbiome balance:

- **Ginger**: Reduces inflammation, promotes motility, and soothes nausea.
- **Peppermint**: Eases bloating, gas, and spasms; also calms the nervous system.
- **Fennel**: Relieves digestive discomfort, including bloating and cramping.
- **Chamomile**: Soothes inflammation in the gut and promotes relaxation.
- **Licorice Root (DGL)**: Protects the gut lining and reduces symptoms of acid reflux or gastritis.

Gut-Lining Protectors

These herbs heal and protect the gut lining, essential for a healthy gut-brain connection:

- **Slippery Elm**: Coats and soothes the GI tract, aiding in conditions like IBS.
- **Marshmallow Root**: Forms a protective layer in the gut and alleviates irritation.
- **Aloe Vera**: Reduces inflammation and promotes healing of the gut lining.

Microbiome Balancers

Certain herbs help restore a healthy balance of gut bacteria:

- **Garlic**: Antimicrobial properties reduce harmful bacteria while promoting beneficial strains.
- **Oregano Oil**: Potent antimicrobial that helps combat gut dysbiosis.
- **Turmeric**: Anti-inflammatory and prebiotic properties support gut health.

Adaptogens for Stress Regulation

Stress negatively affects the gut-brain axis, and adaptogens help regulate the body's stress response:

- **Ashwagandha**: Calms the nervous system, supports adrenal health, and reduces cortisol levels.
- **Holy Basil (Tulsi)**: Promotes relaxation and reduces the impact of stress on digestion.
- **Rhodiola Rosea**: Balances mood and enhances resilience to stress.
- **Panax Ginseng**: Boosts energy while reducing stress and inflammation.

Nervous System Calming Herbs

These herbs soothe the mind and body, promoting better communication along the gut-brain axis:

- **Valerian Root**: Calms the nervous system and promotes restful sleep.

- **Passionflower**: Enhances GABA levels for relaxation and anxiety reduction.
- **Lemon Balm**: Eases tension and promotes a sense of calm.

Inflammation Modulators

Chronic inflammation disrupts the gut-brain axis, and these herbs help reduce it:

- **Turmeric (Curcumin)**: Anti-inflammatory properties benefit both the gut and the brain.
- **Boswellia**: Reduces gut inflammation and supports overall digestive health.
- **Ginger**: Decreases systemic inflammation and improves gut motility.

Brewing the perfect cup of herbal tea

To maximize the potency of your tea, use fresh herbs whenever possible. Start by boiling water, then let it cool for about a minute before pouring over your herbs. This prevents delicate compounds from being destroyed by excessively hot water. Steep for five to ten minutes, depending on the desired strength. For chamomile and fennel, aim for the longer side to extract their full benefits.

While herbal teas are generally safe, it's important to be mindful of potential interactions and contraindications. Some herbs can interact with medications, affecting their efficacy or causing unwanted side effects. For example, chamomile can interact with blood thinners, so consult a healthcare provider if you're on medication. Pregnant women should also exercise caution, as some herbs aren't recommended during pregnancy. Always start with small amounts to see how your body reacts, and gradually increase if everything feels right.

Creating your own herbal tea blends can also be beneficial. For relaxation, try combining lavender and lemon balm. If digestion is your focus, peppermint and licorice root make a dynamic duo. Peppermint soothes the stomach, while licorice root offers additional digestive support. Blend equal parts of each herb and steep as usual. Experiment with proportions to suit your taste and health goals.

Here's a collection of herbal tea recipes that support the brain-gut axis. These recipes use ingredients that promote gut health, reduce stress, and enhance overall well-being.

HERBAL TEA RECIPES

Chamomile Relaxation Tea

- **Ingredients:**
    1. 1 tablespoon dried chamomile flowers (or 1 chamomile tea bag)
    2. 1 teaspoon honey (optional)
    3. 1 cup hot water
- **Instructions:**
    1. Place chamomile flowers in a teapot or mug.
    2. Pour hot water over the flowers and steep for 5-7 minutes.
    3. Strain (if using loose flowers) and add honey if desired.
    4. Sip slowly to relax before bedtime.

Peppermint Digestion Booster

- **Ingredients:**
    1. 1 tablespoon dried peppermint leaves (or 1 peppermint tea bag)
    2. 1-2 slices of fresh ginger (optional)
    3. 1 cup hot water
- **Instructions:**
    1. Add peppermint leaves and ginger to a teapot or mug.
    2. Pour hot water and steep for 5-10 minutes.
    3. Strain (if using loose leaves) and enjoy after meals.

Ginger-Turmeric Immune Tea

- **Ingredients:**
    1. 1 teaspoon grated fresh ginger
    2. 1 teaspoon grated fresh turmeric (or ½ teaspoon ground turmeric)
    3. 1 pinch black pepper
    4. 1 teaspoon honey or lemon juice (optional)
    5. 1.5 cups water
- **Instructions:**
    1. Bring water to a boil and add ginger and turmeric.
    2. Simmer for 10 minutes, then strain into a mug.
    3. Add black pepper (essential for curcumin absorption) and honey or lemon juice.
    4. Enjoy a warm cup, morning or evening.

Green Tea Antioxidant Elixir

- **Ingredients:**
    1. 1 green tea bag or 1 teaspoon loose green tea leaves
    2. 1 teaspoon lemon juice

3. 1 teaspoon honey
4. 1 cup hot water
- **Instructions:**
    1. Brew green tea in hot water (steep for 2-3 minutes to avoid bitterness).
    2. Add lemon juice and honey.
    3. Stir well and sip mid-morning.

Lavender and Lemon Balm Stress Relief Tea

- **Ingredients:**
    1. 1 teaspoon dried lavender buds
    2. 1 teaspoon dried lemon balm leaves
    3. 1 teaspoon honey (optional)
    4. 1 cup hot water
- **Instructions:**
    1. Combine lavender and lemon balm in a teapot or mug.
    2. Pour hot water over the herbs and steep for 5-8 minutes.
    3. Strain and add honey if desired.
    4. Drink in the evening for calmness.

Dandelion Root Detox Tea

- **Ingredients:**
    1. 1 tablespoon roasted dandelion root (available in health stores)
    2. 1.5 cups water
    3. 1 teaspoon honey (optional)
- **Instructions:**
    1. Simmer dandelion root in water for 10 minutes.
    2. Strain into a mug and add honey if preferred.
    3. Drink in the morning to support liver and gut health.

Ashwagandha Adaptogen Tea

- **Ingredients:**
    1. 1 teaspoon ashwagandha powder
    2. 1 teaspoon honey or cinnamon (optional)
    3. 1 cup hot almond or oat milk
- **Instructions:**
    1. Mix ashwagandha powder into hot almond or oat milk.
    2. Stir well and add honey or cinnamon for flavor.
    3. Enjoy in the evening to reduce stress.

Rooibos Vanilla Bliss

- **Ingredients:**
    1. 1 rooibos tea bag or 1 teaspoon loose rooibos leaves
    2. ½ teaspoon vanilla extract
    3. 1 teaspoon honey or maple syrup
    4. 1 cup hot water
- **Instructions:**
    1. Brew rooibos tea in hot water for 5-7 minutes.
    2. Add vanilla extract and honey.
    3. Stir and sip for a caffeine-free antioxidant boost.

Fennel and Mint Digestive Tea

- **Ingredients:**
    1. 1 teaspoon fennel seeds
    2. 1 teaspoon dried mint leaves
    3. 1 cup hot water
- **Instructions:**
    1. Lightly crush fennel seeds.
    2. Combine fennel and mint in a teapot.
    3. Pour hot water and steep for 10 minutes.

4. Strain and drink after meals.

Licorice Root Gut Soother

- **Ingredients:**
    1. 1 teaspoon dried licorice root
    2. 1 teaspoon grated fresh ginger (optional)
    3. 1 cup hot water
- **Instructions:**
    1. Add licorice root and ginger to a teapot.
    2. Pour hot water and steep for 7-10 minutes.
    3. Strain and enjoy when experiencing gut discomfort.

Golden Milk (Turmeric Latte)

- **Ingredients:**
    1. 1 teaspoon turmeric powder
    2. ½ teaspoon cinnamon
    3. 1 cup warm coconut or almond milk
    4. 1 teaspoon honey
    5. 1 pinch black pepper
- **Instructions:**
    1. Heat the milk gently in a saucepan (do not boil).
    2. Stir in turmeric, cinnamon, black pepper, and honey.
    3. Whisk until smooth and frothy.
    4. Pour into a mug and drink as an evening treat.

Gut-Brain Harmony Tea Blend

- **Ingredients:**
    1. 1 teaspoon dried chamomile
    2. 1 teaspoon dried lavender
    3. 1 teaspoon lemon balm

    4. 1 cup hot water
- **Instructions:**
    1. Combine chamomile, lavender, and lemon balm in a teapot.
    2. Pour hot water and steep for 5-7 minutes.
    3. Strain and enjoy as a relaxing gut-brain support tea.

CUSTOMIZING RECIPES

While the recipes are actual and based on established knowledge, herbal effects can vary by individual. To verify their efficacy for personal use:

- Use reputable sources for herbs (e.g., organic or well-reviewed suppliers).
- Adjust the ingredients or dosages to match specific health needs.
- Consult a qualified herbalist or healthcare provider if you have specific medical conditions or concerns.

Digestive Harmony Tea

- **Ingredients:**
    1. 1 teaspoon fennel seeds (supports digestion and reduces bloating)
    2. 1 teaspoon dried peppermint leaves (soothes the gut)
    3. 1 teaspoon dried ginger root (reduces inflammation and supports motility)
    4. 1 cup boiling water
- **Instructions:**
    1. Combine all ingredients in a teapot or mug.
    2. Pour boiling water over the herbs and steep for 7-10 minutes.

3. Strain and sip slowly after meals.

Anti-Inflammatory Microbiome Blend

- **Ingredients:**
    1. 1 teaspoon turmeric powder (anti-inflammatory)
    2. 1 teaspoon cinnamon (stabilizes blood sugar and supports digestion)
    3. 1 pinch black pepper (enhances turmeric absorption)
    4. 1 cup almond milk (optional for a creamy texture)
- **Instructions:**
    1. Heat the milk or water and add the turmeric, cinnamon, and black pepper.
    2. Simmer for 5 minutes, then strain into a cup.
    3. Add a touch of honey or maple syrup if desired.

Prebiotic Power Tea

- **Ingredients:**
    1. 1 teaspoon dried **dandelion** root (rich in prebiotic fibers)
    2. 1 teaspoon chicory root (supports beneficial gut bacteria)
    3. 1 teaspoon dried peppermint leaves (calms the digestive system)
    4. 1.5 cups boiling water
- **Instructions:**
    1. Simmer dandelion and chicory root in water for 10 minutes.
    2. Add peppermint leaves and steep for another 5 minutes.
    3. Strain and enjoy warm.

Gut-Calming Chamomile-Calendula Tea

- **Ingredients:**
    1. 1 teaspoon dried chamomile flowers (anti-inflammatory and soothing)
    2. 1 teaspoon dried calendula flowers (heals and protects gut lining)
    3. 1 teaspoon lemon balm (reduces stress and supports gut-brain connection)
    4. 1 cup boiling water
- **Instructions:**
    1. Combine the herbs in a mug or teapot.
    2. Pour boiling water over the mixture and steep for 8-10 minutes.
    3. Strain and sip before bedtime.

Herbal Detox Tea

- **Ingredients:**
    1. 1 teaspoon dried nettle leaves (detoxifying and nutrient-dense)
    2. 1 teaspoon dried oregano (antimicrobial and supports gut health)
    3. 1 teaspoon dried parsley (natural diuretic and gut-friendly)
    4. 1.5 cups boiling water
- **Instructions:**
    1. Combine the herbs in a pot and simmer in boiling water for 10 minutes.
    2. Strain and serve warm or chilled.

Fermentation Booster Tea

- **Ingredients:**
    1. 1 teaspoon rooibos tea leaves (antioxidant-rich and gut-friendly)
    2. 1 teaspoon dried hibiscus flowers (supports beneficial gut bacteria)
    3. 1 teaspoon orange peel (contains gut-nourishing polyphenols)
    4. 1 cup boiling water
- **Instructions:**
    1. Combine all ingredients in a teapot or infuser.
    2. Steep in boiling water for 5-7 minutes.
    3. Strain and enjoy hot or iced.

Soothing Licorice-Cardamom Tea

- **Ingredients:**
    1. 1 teaspoon dried licorice root (supports gut lining and reduces inflammation)
    2. 3-4 cardamom pods (aids digestion and reduces bloating)
    3. 1 teaspoon dried peppermint leaves (soothes the gut)
    4. 1 cup boiling water
- **Instructions:**
    1. Crush cardamom pods lightly.
    2. Combine licorice root, cardamom, and peppermint in a teapot.
    3. Pour boiling water over the mixture and steep for 7-10 minutes.
    4. Strain and sip after meals.

Immune-Gut Connection Tea

- **Ingredients:**
    1. 1 teaspoon dried echinacea (boosts immunity and gut health)
    2. 1 teaspoon dried elderberries (antioxidant-rich and antimicrobial)
    3. 1 teaspoon grated fresh ginger (reduces inflammation and supports gut motility)
    4. 1 cup boiling water
- **Instructions:**
    1. Simmer echinacea and elderberries in boiling water for 10 minutes.
    2. Add grated ginger and steep for another 5 minutes.
    3. Strain and drink warm.

Caffeine-Free Adaptogen Tea

- **Ingredients:**
    1. 1 teaspoon ashwagandha powder (reduces stress and supports gut-brain axis)
    2. 1 teaspoon dried tulsi (holy basil) leaves (adaptogen and anti-inflammatory)
    3. 1 teaspoon honey (optional)
    4. 1 cup hot almond or oat milk
- **Instructions:**
    1. Mix ashwagandha and tulsi leaves with the hot milk.
    2. Let steep for 5 minutes, then strain.
    3. Add honey for sweetness and enjoy in the evening.

Berry-Gut Antioxidant Tea

- **Ingredients:**
    1. 1 teaspoon dried blueberries or goji berries (rich in polyphenols)
    2. 1 teaspoon hibiscus flowers (balances gut microbiota)
    3. 1 teaspoon green tea leaves (if caffeine is suitable for you)
    4. 1 cup boiling water
- **Instructions:**
    1. Combine all ingredients and steep in boiling water for 5-7 minutes.
    2. Strain and enjoy hot or cold.

Tips for Preparation:

- **Use Quality Ingredients:** Choose organic herbs and roots to avoid pesticides that could harm gut bacteria.
- **Steeping Time:** Adjust the steeping time based on the herb, as over-brewing can make some teas bitter.
- **Drink Regularly:** Enjoy 1–2 cups daily for consistent microbiome support.

Feel free to research the individual components of each of these plants, tea leaves, and flowers—you'll be pleasantly surprised. Let's take a look at the **dandelions**, for example. An article published by Total Balanced Health talks about how the dandelion's "greens (leaves) and roots alike carry several major health benefits. High in fiber to help you stay regular, dandelion leaves also serve as a mild diuretic, which can help with fluid retention from PMS or urination difficulty caused by bladder infections.

Dandelion leaves are a great source of vitamin K, important for blood clotting, with 535% of the U.S. RDA per cup of greens. One cup (around 55 grams) of dandelion greens contains approximately **428–535 micrograms of vitamin K**. The U.S. Recommended Dietary Allowance (RDA) for vitamin K is **90 micrograms per day for women** and **120 micrograms per day for men**. Therefore, it provides more than 5 times the recommended daily allowance of vitamin K for an average adult. Since long-term use of antibiotics can lead to a vitamin K deficiency, dandelion greens are an excellent choice post-treatment. Just wait until your course of antibiotics is complete before eating too many, as dandelion may impede the absorption of antibiotics into your bloodstream.

You'll discover one cup of raw dandelion greens provides a complete 112% of your daily RDA of vitamin A, which is vital for healthy bones, keen eyesight, and a strong immune system. They pack in nearly a third of your daily RDA in vitamins C, E, B2, and B6. Plus, they're rich in minerals, including calcium, iron, manganese, potassium, magnesium, and boron (which raises blood levels of estrogen to help preserve bone strength).

Vegetarians and vegans will be happy to learn that dandelions are high in protein, with essential amino acids comparable to or better than red meat, poultry, and eggs. And like most healthy greens, dandelion leaves are diet-friendly, weighing in at only 25 calories per cup.

Oregano tea, made from the leaves of the oregano plant (*Origanum vulgare*), is also known for its medicinal properties. It has a high content of antioxidants, vitamins, and compounds like thymol, carvacrol, and rosmarinic acid. These compounds contribute to its antimicrobial, anti-inflammatory, and digestive benefits.

Benefits of Oregano Tea

1. **Supports Gut Health:**
   - Oregano has antibacterial and antifungal properties, helping maintain a balanced gut microbiota.
   - It can reduce bloating, gas, and indigestion by aiding digestion and combating harmful pathogens in the gut.
2. **Boosts Immunity:**
   - Rich in antioxidants and compounds like thymol and carvacrol, oregano tea can help strengthen the immune system and fight off infections.
3. **Anti-inflammatory Properties:**
   - Oregano contains rosmarinic acid, which can reduce inflammation in the body, benefiting conditions like arthritis or inflammatory bowel issues.
4. **Relieves Respiratory Issues:**
   - Oregano tea is often used as a natural remedy for coughs, colds, and sinus congestion due to its expectorant properties.
   - It may help clear mucus and soothe sore throats.
5. **Promotes Mental Clarity and Relaxation:**
   - Oregano's essential oils can have a mild calming effect, reducing stress and supporting the brain-gut axis.
6. **Rich in Nutrients:**
   - Contains vitamins A, C, and E, as well as iron, manganese, and calcium, which contribute to overall wellness.
7. **Antimicrobial Effects:**
   - The tea's antibacterial and antifungal compounds can help combat infections, including candida and other gut-related pathogens.

How to Make Oregano Tea

Basic Recipe:

- **Ingredients:**
    1. 1 tablespoon fresh oregano leaves (or 1 teaspoon dried leaves)
    2. 1 cup boiling water
    3. Optional: Honey or lemon for flavor.
- **Instructions:**
    1. Rinse the oregano leaves (if fresh) to remove any dirt.
    2. Place the leaves in a teapot or mug.
    3. Pour boiling water over the leaves and cover.
    4. Steep for 5-10 minutes, depending on desired strength.
    5. Strain and add honey or lemon if desired.
    6. Enjoy warm, sipping slowly.

Enhanced Recipes:

1. **Oregano-Ginger Tea for Digestion:**
    - Add a few slices of fresh ginger to the tea while steeping.
    - Benefits: Combines oregano's gut-balancing properties with ginger's anti-nausea effects.
2. **Oregano-Lemon Tea for Immunity:**
    - Add 1 tablespoon fresh lemon juice and a pinch of turmeric to the prepared tea.
    - Benefits: Boosts antioxidant and anti-inflammatory effects.
3. **Oregano-Mint Tea for Relaxation:**
    - Add 1 teaspoon dried mint leaves to oregano leaves during steeping.

- Benefits: Enhances the calming and digestive properties of the tea.
4. **Oregano-Honey Tea for Respiratory Relief:**
   - Add 1 teaspoon raw honey to the tea.
   - Benefits: Soothes sore throats and enhances oregano's antimicrobial effects.

Precautions and Side Effects

- **Allergic Reactions:** People allergic to mint-family plants (e.g., basil, thyme, mint) may experience reactions.
- **Pregnancy and Breastfeeding:** Large amounts of oregano tea should be avoided, as oregano can stimulate uterine contractions.
- **Drug Interactions:** Oregano tea may interact with blood-thinning medications or those for diabetes and blood pressure.
- **Excessive Use:** Overconsumption can lead to mild stomach upset.

ESSENTIAL OILS AND THE GUT-BRAIN AXIS

Essential oils are concentrated plant extracts known for their therapeutic properties. Through aromatherapy or topical application, these oils interact with the limbic system in the brain, which controls emotions and stress responses. By calming the nervous system and reducing stress, essential oils can indirectly benefit gut health. Stress is a major disruptor of the gut-brain axis, often causing digestive issues like bloating, cramps, or even irritable bowel syndrome (IBS).

CALMING AND STRESS-REDUCING ESSENTIAL OILS

These oils help reduce stress and anxiety, which are key contributors to gut dysfunction.

Lavender (*Lavandula angustifolia*)

- **Benefits:** Calms the nervous system, reduces anxiety, promotes restful sleep.
- **Uses:** Diffuse before bed or apply diluted oil to pulse points.

Chamomile (*Matricaria chamomilla* or *Chamaemelum nobile*)

- **Benefits:** Eases tension, soothes digestive discomfort caused by stress.
- **Uses:** Add to a warm bath or mix with carrier oil for abdominal massage.

Bergamot (*Citrus bergamia*)

- **Benefits:** Uplifts mood, reduces cortisol levels, and calms the mind.
- **Uses:** Diffuse during the day or apply diluted to the chest.

Ylang Ylang (*Cananga odorata*)

- **Benefits:** Promotes relaxation, reduces anxiety, and balances emotions.
- **Uses:** Inhale directly or use in a massage blend.

Rose (*Rosa damascena*)

- **Benefits:** Alleviates emotional distress, fosters feelings of calm and comfort.
- **Uses:** Add to a diffuser or dab diluted oil on the wrists.

DIGESTIVE-SUPPORTING ESSENTIAL OILS

These oils can directly benefit gut health by reducing bloating, cramps, and digestive discomfort.

Peppermint (*Mentha × piperita*)

- **Benefits:** Relieves bloating and indigestion; calms digestive muscles.
- **Uses:** Apply diluted oil to the abdomen or inhale after meals.

Ginger (*Zingiber officinale*)

- **Benefits:** Reduces nausea, enhances gut motility, and alleviates inflammation.
- **Uses:** Add a few drops to a warm compress for abdominal use or diffuse.

Fennel (*Foeniculum vulgare*)

- **Benefits:** Eases bloating and gas; promotes smooth digestion.
- **Uses:** Apply diluted oil to the stomach area in circular motions.

Cardamom (*Elettaria cardamomum*)

- **Benefits:** Soothes the stomach and supports healthy digestion.
- **Uses:** Diffuse or use as part of a massage blend for the abdomen.

Lemongrass (*Cymbopogon citratus*)

- **Benefits:** Aids digestion and has mild stress-relieving properties.
- **Uses:** Diffuse during meals or combine with carrier oil for topical application.

MOOD-ENHANCING AND GUT-BRAIN AXIS OILS

These oils help modulate emotions and reduce stress, which can positively impact gut-brain communication.

Frankincense (*Boswellia carterii*)

- **Benefits:** Supports relaxation and emotional grounding; reduces inflammation.
- **Uses:** Diffuse during meditation or mix with carrier oil for topical use.

Clary Sage (*Salvia sclarea*)

- **Benefits:** Balances hormones and mood; promotes deep relaxation.
- **Uses:** Diffuse or add to bathwater for a calming soak.

Sweet Orange (*Citrus sinensis*)

- **Benefits:** Boosts mood, reduces anxiety, and enhances gut motility.
- **Uses:** Diffuse during stressful periods or add a few drops to a carrier oil for massage.

Patchouli (*Pogostemon cablin*)

- **Benefits:** Balances emotions, alleviates stress, and reduces digestive issues.
- **Uses:** Use in a diffuser or as part of a calming massage blend.

Cedarwood (*Cedrus atlantica*)

- **Benefits:** Grounds emotions, reduces tension, and supports relaxation.
- **Uses:** Add to a diffuser or apply diluted to the soles of the feet.

IMMUNE-BOOSTING AND ANTI-INFLAMMATORY ESSENTIAL OILS

These oils support overall health, which indirectly benefits gut function.

Tea Tree (*Melaleuca alternifolia*)

- **Benefits:** Antimicrobial properties support a balanced microbiome.
- **Uses:** Diffuse to purify the air or apply diluted to the skin.

Eucalyptus (*Eucalyptus globulus*)

- **Benefits:** Reduces inflammation and improves respiratory health, aiding stress relief.
- **Uses:** Inhale deeply or use in steam inhalation.

Lemon (*Citrus limon*)

- **Benefits:** Cleanses the body and supports the immune system.
- **Uses:** Diffuse during the day for a refreshing atmosphere.

BLENDS AND RECIPES

Stress-Soothing Diffuser Blend:

- 3 drops lavender
- 2 drops chamomile
- 2 drops bergamot

Digestive Support Massage Oil:

- 2 drops fennel
- 2 drops peppermint
- 1 drop ginger
- 1 tablespoon carrier oil (e.g., coconut or almond)

Mood Uplifting Diffuser Blend:

- 3 drops sweet orange
- 2 drops ylang ylang
- 1 drop frankincense

Relaxing Bath Soak:

- 5 drops clary sage
- 3 drops cedarwood
- 2 tablespoons Epsom salt

Tips for Safe Use:

1. **Dilution:** Always dilute essential oils in a carrier oil (e.g., coconut, jojoba) before applying to the skin.
2. **Patch Test:** Conduct a patch test for allergies before use.
3. **Avoid Ingestion:** Essential oils should not be ingested unless guided by a healthcare professional.
4. **Pregnancy Caution:** Consult a doctor before using oils like clary sage or fennel during pregnancy.

SUPPLEMENTS FOR GUT-BRAIN WELLNESS

Supplements offer a convenient way to fill nutritional gaps that diet alone might not cover. When it comes to gut-brain wellness, certain supplements like Omega-3 are known for their anti-inflammatory effects. These fatty acids, often derived from fish oil, help reduce inflammation throughout the body, including the gut and brain. So, if you are not eating enough foods rich in Omega-3 fatty acids, consider taking supplements.

When it comes to choosing the right supplement, look for products that have undergone third-party testing to ensure quality and safety. Understanding ingredient labels is also crucial. Avoid products with unnecessary fillers or artificial additives; instead, look for those that offer pure, active ingredients. It's important to remember that supplements are just that—supplementary to a healthy diet and lifestyle. They are not a cure-all but can offer significant support when used correctly.

Before starting any supplement, consider potential interactions with medications or existing health conditions. Consulting with a healthcare provider can help identify any risks. Some individuals may have allergies or sensitivities to certain herbal products or compounds found in supplements. For example, those with fish allergies should avoid omega-3 supplements derived from fish oil, opting instead for plant-based alternatives like flaxseed oil.

INCORPORATING ADAPTOGENS

Adaptogens are a group of herbs that help your body handle stress and stay balanced. When life gets overwhelming, adaptogens help control your body's response by keeping stress hormones like cortisol in check, reducing the strain stress puts on you.

They work by balancing the hypothalamic-pituitary-adrenal (HPA) axis, which is the system in your body that controls how you respond to stress. This system also regulates important functions like digestion, your immune system, and how your body uses energy. By keeping the HPA axis in harmony, adaptogens help your body perform at its best, even when life is stressful.

Among the most popular adaptogens, ashwagandha reduces cortisol and alleviates anxiety. Rhodiola can enhance energy and mental clarity, making it ideal for those midday slumps when focus and concentration fade. Holy basil, known for reducing stress-induced inflammation, brings peace and balance. These adaptogens offer unique benefits, but their collective power is truly transformative.

Incorporating adaptogens into your daily routine is easy, start by taking between 300 mg to 500 mg per day, and adjust based on how your body responds. Adaptogens come in various forms—powders, capsules, and teas. Powders can be blended into smoothies, capsules offer a quick and easy option, and teas provide a calming ritual to your day. Timing is crucial; for instance, ashwagandha is best taken in the evening due to its calming effects, while Rhodiola should be consumed in the morning to boost energy and clarity.

Combining adaptogens with other herbs can enhance their benefits. Pairing ashwagandha with chamomile can help both stress and digestion. By combining different adaptogens, you can tailor blends to support your specific needs.

Embracing adaptogens as part of your wellness routine can transform how you handle stress, providing a natural way to enhance resilience, boost energy, and maintain a balanced state of mind.

THE MICROBIOME'S ROLE IN MENTAL HEALTH

The bacteria in your gut do more than just help with digestion—they also play a role in your mood and mental health. Recent research shows that these tiny organisms can have a significant impact, especially on conditions like PTSD. When you go through something traumatic, it doesn't just affect your mind; it can also upset the balance of your gut bacteria. Trauma can change the gut's bacteria and trigger inflammation in your body, which can make PTSD symptoms worse.

PTSD AND GUT BACTERIA: HEALING TRAUMA FROM WITHIN

The link between PTSD and the gut microbiome is a growing area of research that's getting a lot of attention. Studies suggest that trauma can change the balance of gut bacteria, which may make PTSD symptoms harder to overcome. After a traumatic event, the gut's bacteria can shift, leading to higher levels of inflammation signals in the body. These signals act like alarms, keeping the body in a constant state of alert, which can worsen stress and anxiety, making recovery more difficult. The gut and brain are closely connected through the gut-brain axis, a communication system that allows the gut to influence emotions and behaviors, sometimes leading to anxiety or depression.

Treatments focusing on the gut microbiome are showing promise in reducing PTSD symptoms. For example, psychobiotics—special probiotics that affect the gut-brain connection—can help rebalance the gut, lower inflammation, and promote emotional stability. The diet also plays a key role in gut health. Eating foods rich in fiber, antioxidants, and probiotics, like fermented foods, can support healthy bacteria in the gut. When combined with practices like yoga and meditation, these approaches can calm both the gut and the mind.

Studies show that restoring a healthy microbiome can reduce anxiety and depression linked to PTSD. Personalized treatment can make interventions even more effective. Since each of our microbiomes is unique, it makes sense to customize probiotics to make treatments more targeted and successful.

OCD: CAN GUT HEALTH OFFER NEW HOPE?

Obsessive-Compulsive Disorder (OCD) is a condition that involves repetitive thoughts and behaviors that can disrupt daily life. While it can be challenging to understand and manage, recent research suggests that the gut microbiome may play a role in OCD. Studies show that people with OCD often have less variety in their gut bacteria compared to those without the condition. This might affect the gut-brain axis because when this connection is disrupted, it contributes to the compulsive behaviors seen in OCD. The gut microbiome might be influencing the brain's chemical signals, creating a cycle that reinforces obsessive thoughts and actions. Although scientists are still studying the exact mechanisms, the connection between gut health and OCD offers hope for those dealing with this condition.

Using gut health as part of OCD treatment is a new area of research. Probiotics are emerging as a potential tool to help restore balance in the gut microbiome. In addition to probiotics, making dietary changes can also support gut and mental health. A fiber-rich diet, prebiotics, and fermented foods can help nourish healthy gut bacteria. This, in turn, might boost the production of neurotransmitters like serotonin, which helps regulate mood and could reduce compulsive urges. These approaches work best as part of a comprehensive treatment plan alongside traditional therapies.

Some studies are exploring the impact of probiotics and dietary changes on OCD symptoms. A study presented at the 2023 International Digestive Disease Forum found that OCD patients had lower bacterial diversity compared to healthy individuals, and animal studies showed that specific probiotic strains, such as *Lactobacillus rhamnosus* GG and *Lactobacillus casei*, could reduce OCD-like behaviors in rodents. Additionally, a 2015 study highlighted by BrainsWay found that probiotics may lower cortisol production, a stress-related hormone often elevated in OCD patients.

While these findings are promising, more extensive clinical trials are necessary to confirm the effectiveness of gut-focused therapies. Nonetheless, these early studies indicate that addressing gut health could offer new avenues for individuals who have not responded well to traditional treatments.

As research continues, scientists are exploring new tools and treatments focused on the microbiome. These tests could help healthcare providers create tailored treatments for each person based on their unique microbiome. Other experimental therapies, like fecal microbiota transplants (transferring healthy gut bacteria from one person to another), are also being studied as possible ways to restore gut balance and improve OCD symptoms. While more research is needed, this area of study offers hope for better, more personalized treatment options in the future.

ANXIETY ALLEVIATION: PROBIOTICS AS A NATURAL REMEDY

Imagine you're feeling anxious, and nothing seems to calm your mind. Two types of bacteria, Lactobacillus and Bifidobacterium, are gaining attention for their calming effects. These probiotics actively communicate with your brain and even influence your skin. This is all part of the gut-brain-skin axis, a system that connects these parts of your body and shows how everything is interconnected. A meta-analysis published in *Gut Pathogens* revealed that interventions using *Lactobacillus* and *Bifidobacterium* strains led to reductions in anxiety symptoms compared to placebos.

Probiotics help reduce anxiety in amazing ways. One way is by increasing levels of GABA, a calming neurotransmitter in your brain. By boosting GABA production, probiotics help your body manage stress, reduce anxiety, and create a sense of calm. It's like having a natural stress-relief system working inside you to keep everything balanced.

Again, for probiotics to thrive in your gut, they need the prebiotics, which feed the good bacteria and help them grow. Using probiotics to reduce anxiety is a great natural approach.

DEPRESSION AND THE GUT: UNRAVELING THE CONNECTION

Our gut might hold the key to understanding depression. Studies show that when the balance of bacteria in the gut is disrupted, dysbiosis can play a major role in causing depressive symptoms. This makes sense because the gut is often called our "second brain," and the connection between the two is stronger than we once thought. Research has found that people with depression often have different gut bacteria compared to those without the condition. This imbalance can cause inflammation, and when the gut is inflamed, it sends distress signals to the brain, disrupting mood regulation and contributing to feelings of sadness or hopelessness.

The way the gut and brain interact is complex but fascinating. The gut can influence the HPA axis, which controls our stress response. When the gut is unbalanced, the HPA axis can become overactive, leading to higher levels of stress hormones that worsen depressive symptoms. The gut also produces much of the body's serotonin, a chemical that helps regulate mood. If the gut's bacteria are out of balance, serotonin production can drop, leading to lower levels of this important mood-boosting chemical. Dopamine, another chemical linked to feelings of motivation and reward, can also be affected by gut health. These processes highlight how closely gut health is tied to mental well-being.

Improving gut health offers a promising way to reduce depressive symptoms. Combining probiotics and prebiotics creates a healthier gut environment that can positively influence mood, and eating foods high in fiber, antioxidants, and omega-3 fatty acids can improve gut health, lower inflammation, and support the production of mood-regulating chemicals, providing a natural way to manage depression.

Recent studies have focused on the impact of probiotics and dietary changes on mood. A pilot randomized clinical trial published in *JAMA Psychiatry* investigated the effects of a multi-strain probiotic supplement as an add-on treatment for patients with major depressive disorder. The study found that participants who received the probiotic showed more significant improvements in depressive and anxiety symptoms compared to those who received a placebo.

Additionally, a meta-analysis in *BMC Psychiatry* evaluated the effects of prebiotics, probiotics, and synbiotics on individuals with depression. The analysis concluded that these interventions significantly improved depressive symptoms compared to placebo treatments. However, subgroup analysis confirmed the significant antidepressant effects primarily for agents containing probiotics.

These findings, along with anecdotal evidence from individuals who have experienced mood improvements through gut-focused therapies, suggest that targeting gut health could be a promising approach to managing depression. However, more extensive and rigorous studies are needed to fully understand these interventions' efficacy.

ADDRESSING SPECIFIC MENTAL HEALTH CONDITIONS

Have you ever wondered why some days it seems impossible to focus? For people with ADHD, this is a daily reality that turns tasks into challenges and thoughts into an incessant buzz. While many factors contribute to ADHD, researchers have uncovered a surprising player—yes, you guessed it, the gut.

ADHD: ENHANCING FOCUS THROUGH GUT OPTIMIZATION

Studies have found links between gut health and ADHD symptoms, suggesting that an imbalanced gut microbiome might contribute to the inattention and hyperactivity characteristic of this condition. Dysbiosis might exacerbate these symptoms. When this balance is disrupted, it leads to inflammation, which is thought to influence cognitive and behavioral symptoms associated with ADHD. By understanding this connection, we can reduce hyperactivity through dietary and lifestyle changes.

Dietary interventions can help manage ADHD symptoms. Again, Omega-3 fatty acids, known for their brain-boosting properties, and probiotic strains like Lactobacillus and Bifidobacterium might help enhance cognitive function. Cutting back on processed foods and sugars is also crucial. These foods can spike blood sugar levels, leading to energy crashes that make ADHD symptoms worse.

For parents and individuals navigating ADHD, practical strategies can make a big difference. Creating weekly menus that include gut-friendly foods ensures a balanced intake of nutrients. Involve your child in the process to make healthy eating more appealing and empower them to take an active role in their health.

Additionally, engaging in mindfulness practices can support focus. Simple techniques like deep breathing exercises or mindful coloring can help calm the mind and improve concentration. These practices encourage a sense of presence, reducing the overwhelming sensations that often accompany ADHD.

Mindful Journaling for Focus

Try keeping a daily journal. At the end of each day, jot down what you ate, your mood, and your ability to focus. Look for patterns, and consider how dietary changes or mindfulness practices might be influencing your attention and hyperactivity.

DEMENTIA: THE GUT'S ROLE IN COGNITIVE HEALTH

Many of us worry about losing mental sharpness as we age, but part of the solution might lie in our gut. Keeping your gut healthy could lower the risk of brain-related conditions like dementia. When the gut is out of balance, it can produce harmful effects on the brain. This happens because gut bacteria create substances called metabolites that travel through your bloodstream to your brain. If the gut is unhealthy, these substances can negatively affect brain function and contribute to mental decline.

Colorful fruits and vegetables are packed with antioxidants and polyphenols, which act like shields for your brain cells. These nutrients fight oxidative stress, which causes damage to cells and contributes to mental decline. Physical activity also plays an important role in keeping both your gut and brain healthy. Exercise encourages the growth of beneficial gut bacteria and improves blood flow to the brain. This increased blood flow supports the creation of new brain cells, boosting mental clarity. So, a simple walk doesn't just strengthen your body—it also helps your mind.

Recent research highlights the Mediterranean diet's potential to reduce the risk of cognitive decline by supporting both gut and brain health. This diet emphasizes plant-based foods, healthy fats like olive oil, and moderate consumption of fish and poultry. Its high content of anti-inflammatory compounds and antioxidants helps maintain a balanced gut microbiome, which in turn supports cognitive function.

A study published in *Frontiers in Nutrition* discusses how the Mediterranean diet, rich in antioxidants, vitamins, and polyphenols, demonstrates neuroprotective potential. These components counteract processes like oxidative stress and inflammation, which are involved in neurodegenerative diseases.

Additionally, a systematic review in the *British Journal of Nutrition* indicates that even short-term adherence to a Mediterranean-style dietary pattern can improve cognition and mood. The review suggests that the diet's benefits might work through quick changes in the body, like improved blood flow to the brain, reduced inflammation, and lower cell damage.

These findings suggest that the Mediterranean diet's emphasis on plant-based foods, healthy fats, and lean proteins can support both gut and brain health, potentially reducing the risk of cognitive decline.

Additionally, staying mentally and socially active is also important for brain health. Activities like puzzles, learning new skills, or socializing with friends help keep your mind sharp and your emotions positive. Consider joining a group or taking part in community activities to stay engaged.

BIPOLAR DISORDER: STABILIZING MOOD WITH NUTRITIONAL INTERVENTIONS

Understanding how gut health relates to mood swings in bipolar disorder provides new ways to manage the condition. What you eat can have a huge impact on stabilizing your mood. Include magnesium and zinc to maintain a healthy balance. Magnesium, found in foods like almonds, spinach, and black beans, helps relax your nervous system and can lessen mood swings. Zinc, found in oysters, beef, and pumpkin seeds, supports brain function and helps balance mood. Foods rich in omega-3 fatty acids also help by reducing inflammation and improving brain health. Dietary changes can help reduce how often and how severely mood swings occur.

Gut-brain therapies incorporating probiotics and prebiotics have also shown promise in treating bipolar disorder. While these dietary and lifestyle changes won't cure bipolar disorder, they offer a helpful way to manage it.

AUTISM SPECTRUM DISORDERS (ASD) AND THE GUT-BRAIN CONNECTION

Autism Spectrum Disorders (ASD) are complex conditions that researchers are still working to fully understand. One area of interest is the connection between gut health and ASD symptoms. In ASD, an imbalance in gut bacteria may influence how the brain processes information, which could contribute to some of the behaviors associated with the disorder.

Research suggests a link between gut microbiota and ASD. Studies have found that individuals with ASD often exhibit distinct gut microbiota profiles compared to neurotypical individuals. For instance, a study published in *Gut Pathogens* observed significant differences in the gut bacteria of children with ASD.

Another study in *Frontiers in Cellular and Infection Microbiology* highlighted that imbalances in gut bacteria might influence neurological development and behavior in ASD. The research suggests that certain gut bacteria can affect the central nervous system, potentially contributing to ASD symptoms.

Additionally, a systematic review in the *International Journal of Molecular Sciences* analyzed various studies and found evidence of gut microbiota alterations in individuals with ASD. The review emphasized the importance of gut health in understanding and potentially managing ASD symptoms.

These studies offer a new perspective on potential therapeutic strategies focusing on gut health. They suggest that restoring balance in the gut microbiome could potentially ease certain symptoms. Supporting gut health through diet and lifestyle changes might provide a new way to manage some aspects of ASD. While more research is needed, this connection opens up new possibilities for helping those with ASD.

PARKINSON'S DISEASE AND GUT HEALTH

Parkinson's Disease, known for causing tremors and movement issues, also has a strong link to gut health. When the gut's balance of bacteria is disrupted, it can trigger a chain reaction that affects the brain. This imbalance, along with a "leaky gut" where harmful substances escape into the bloodstream, can cause neuroinflammation (inflammation in the brain), which is closely tied to Parkinson's Disease.

The gut might be sending distress signals that speed up the progression of the disease. Supporting gut health by including probiotics (beneficial bacteria) and prebiotics (foods that feed good bacteria) in your diet could help reduce inflammation and protect against some of these processes. Improving gut health is showing promise as a way to complement traditional treatments and slow down the effects of Parkinson's.

NATURAL APPROACH FOR AUTOIMMUNE CONDITIONS

The gut is a key player in autoimmune conditions, even though its role is often overlooked. As we already know, dysbiosis causes chronic inflammation, which is the culprit in many autoimmune diseases. This inflammation often leads to the development and worsening of these conditions. Understanding the connection between inflammation and the gut is important for anyone exploring natural ways to support their autoimmune condition.

UNDERSTANDING GUT HEALTH AND INFLAMMATION

The connection between the gut and inflammation works like a chain reaction—one small problem can trigger a series of events that lead to chronic inflammation. When the gut becomes unbalanced, its lining can become "leaky," which means it no longer acts as the strong barrier it's supposed to be. Instead, it allows harmful substances like toxins, bacteria, and undigested food particles to pass into the bloodstream. The immune system sees these as threats and overreacts, leading to widespread inflammation. This chronic inflammation is a key factor in many autoimmune diseases.

Dysbiosis, the imbalance in gut bacteria, makes things even worse. When the gut's ecosystem of bacteria is thrown off balance, immune signaling goes haywire, increasing the risk of inflammation and autoimmune diseases. It is important to emphasize that the gut doesn't just react to problems; it actively influences how the immune system works, often triggering or worsening autoimmune conditions.

The immune system and gut health are closely linked through a part of the gut called gut-associated lymphoid tissue (GALT). This tissue helps the immune system decide how to respond to substances that enter the body. Depending on the balance of gut bacteria, they can either calm the immune system or trigger inflammation. So, keeping this system healthy is a great way to prevent unnecessary inflammation.

Inflammation in autoimmune diseases often starts in the gut. One major process involved is cytokine production. Cytokines are molecules that help regulate immune responses, but when too many are produced, they cause chronic inflammation. Gut bacteria play a big role in this process because dysbiosis can lead to an overproduction of cytokines. This triggers a cycle of inflammation that can cause autoimmune flare-ups, where the immune system attacks the body's own tissues.

Doctors often look at inflammatory markers to understand the body's level of inflammation. Two common markers are C-reactive protein (CRP) and erythrocyte sedimentation rate (ESR). High levels of CRP are a warning sign of underlying issues. ESR measures how quickly red blood cells settle in a test tube, and when they do so quickly, it's a sign of inflammation.

A meta-analysis published in the *American Journal of Clinical Pathology* evaluated the diagnostic accuracy of ESR and CRP in detecting acute inflammation. The study found that both markers have similar diagnostic accuracy, especially in orthopedic conditions, and that using both ESR and CRP together can yield higher diagnostic accuracy.

Another review article in the *WMJ* discussed the clinical utility of ESR and CRP, highlighting that while both tests are influenced by various factors, they provide valuable information when used in conjunction with clinical history and physical examination.

By keeping the gut balanced, you can help regulate immune responses and reduce the chronic inflammation that drives autoimmune diseases.

FOOD VS. AUTOIMMUNE CONDITIONS

Supporting and managing autoimmune conditions often starts with an **anti-inflammatory diet**. This means focusing on whole, natural foods instead of processed ones. Colorful vegetables, fruits, and lean proteins are packed with nutrients like vitamins, minerals, and fiber that processed foods lack. By choosing fresh, unprocessed options, you can avoid additives and preservatives that can worsen inflammation. Instead of just cutting out harmful foods, this diet focuses on adding nourishing options to your meals.

One key part of this diet is balancing omega-3 and omega-6 fatty acids, which are important for controlling inflammation. Omega-6 fats, found in many oils and processed foods, can promote inflammation. On the other hand, omega-3 fats, found in foods like fatty fish (salmon, mackerel, sardines), flaxseeds, and walnuts, are anti-inflammatory and help keep your body in balance. Eating more omega-3s while reducing omega-6s can make a big difference in your overall health.

ANTI-INFLAMMATORY FOODS TO INCLUDE:

Fruits

1. **Berries** (blueberries, strawberries, raspberries, blackberries)
2. **Citrus fruits** (oranges, lemons, limes, grapefruit)
3. **Cherries** (especially tart cherries)
4. **Pineapple** (contains bromelain)
5. **Apples**
6. **Papaya**

Vegetables

1. **Leafy greens** (spinach, kale, Swiss chard)
2. **Broccoli**
3. **Cauliflower**
4. **Brussels sprouts**
5. **Beets**
6. **Carrots**
7. **Bell peppers**
8. **Sweet potatoes**

Healthy Fats

1. **Olive oil** (extra virgin)
2. **Avocados**
3. **Nuts** (almonds, walnuts)
4. **Seeds** (chia seeds, flaxseeds, sunflower seeds)
5. **Fatty fish** (salmon, mackerel, sardines, tuna, herring)

6. **Coconut oil** (in moderation)

Whole Grains and Legumes

1. **Oats**
2. **Quinoa**
3. **Brown rice**
4. **Lentils**
5. **Chickpeas**

Spices and Herbs

1. **Turmeric** (curcumin is the active ingredient; pair with black pepper for better absorption)
2. **Ginger**
3. **Garlic**
4. **Cinnamon**
5. **Rosemary**
6. **Thyme**

Fermented Foods

1. **Yogurt** (with live cultures)
2. **Kefir**
3. **Kimchi**
4. **Sauerkraut**
5. **Miso**

Beverages

1. **Green tea** (rich in antioxidants like EGCG)
2. **Chamomile tea**
3. **Turmeric tea**

4. Bone broth
5. Water infused with lemon or cucumber

Other Foods

1. **Dark chocolate** (70% or higher cocoa content)
2. **Tomatoes** (especially cooked, as they release lycopene)
3. **Mushrooms** (shiitake, maitake, reishi)
4. **Basil seeds**
5. **Seaweed**

Dietary Patterns to Follow

1. **The Mediterranean Diet**: This diet focuses on plant-based foods, healthy fats like olive oil, and lean proteins such as fish and poultry. It's a balanced approach that includes fruits, vegetables, whole grains, and nuts while also encouraging you to enjoy meals slowly. It's not just healthy, it's delicious and sustainable.
2. **The Autoimmune Protocol (AIP)**: AIP is an elimination diet that temporarily removes foods like grains, dairy, and legumes, which can trigger inflammation. After a reset period, foods are reintroduced gradually to identify specific triggers.

Making It Work for You

Incorporating anti-inflammatory foods into your diet can be simple and enjoyable. Start with easy recipes like turmeric-spiced lentil soup, berry smoothies, and roasted vegetables paired with grilled salmon.

Meal prepping can help keep you on track. Spend some time each week cooking large batches of healthy meals, like roasted veggies or baked salmon, so you have quick, nutritious options ready to go.

NATURAL REMEDIES FOR AUTOIMMUNE SYMPTOM RELIEF

When managing autoimmune symptoms, natural remedies like herbs, essential oils, and lifestyle changes can provide support. For example, aloe vera can be taken to calm inflammation in the digestive system. Another helpful supplement is Boswellia extract, made from the resin of the Boswellia tree. Known for relieving joint pain and stiffness, it's a natural alternative to over-the-counter painkillers, reducing inflammation without harsh side effects. Regular use of Boswellia can improve mobility and ease discomfort, making it especially beneficial for conditions like rheumatoid arthritis.

Essential oils can also help with managing autoimmune symptoms. For instance, lavender oil has anti-inflammatory properties, so adding a few drops to a diffuser can help. Similarly, frankincense oil, often called the "king of oils," can help with joint pain and swelling. You can apply it to your skin or inhale it to promote relaxation and ease stress, which is a common trigger for autoimmune flare-ups.

Lifestyle changes are just as important in managing symptoms. Stress-reducing activities like yoga and tai chi can make a big difference. These exercises help calm your mind while improving flexibility and strength. Even light exercise boosts blood flow, improves your mood, and benefits your overall health. Getting enough sleep is equally important. During sleep, your body repairs itself, restores energy, and heals tissues. Prioritizing quality rest helps your body stay strong and better manage autoimmune symptoms.

Other complementary therapies, like acupuncture and chiropractic care, also offer relief. Many people with autoimmune conditions find that acupuncture helps reduce flare-ups and provides long-term symptom relief. Chiropractic adjustments can improve communication between your brain and body, potentially reducing pain.

Together, these natural remedies—herbal supplements, essential oils, stress-reducing activities, and complementary therapies—offer more than just symptom relief. They enable you to take charge of your health by supporting your body's natural healing processes. This holistic approach provides a pathway to managing autoimmune symptoms and building a healthier lifestyle.

OTHER CONDITIONS DIRECTLY ASSOCIATED WITH GUT HEALTH

Three chapters of this book address diseases and conditions that have some relation and are affected by the gut-brain connection. While most of them have very similar recommendations for improvement, it was important to break them down individually to show each connection. Understanding these conditions helps you see how vital gut health is to overall well-being.

Menopause and the Gut-Brain Connection

Menopause has a significant relationship with the gut-brain connection.

Hormonal Changes Impact Gut Health

During menopause, levels of estrogen and progesterone decrease. These hormones play an important role in maintaining a healthy gut lining and supporting a balanced gut microbiome. Lower levels of these hormones can lead to:

- **Gut dysbiosis**: An imbalance in gut bacteria, which may cause digestive issues like bloating, constipation, or diarrhea.
- **Increased intestinal permeability**: Also known as "leaky gut," this can lead to inflammation and a heightened immune response.

Gut Microbiome Influences Hormonal Regulation

The gut microbiome helps regulate hormones, including estrogen, through a collection of bacteria called the estrobolome. These bacteria process and regulate circulating estrogens. When the gut microbiome is imbalanced, it can disrupt estrogen metabolism, potentially worsening menopause symptoms like mood swings, hot flashes, and fatigue.

Gut-Brain Axis Affects Mood and Mental Health

The gut-brain axis, the communication network between the gut and the brain, plays a major role in mood and cognitive health. During menopause, hormonal changes can lead to:

- **Increased stress and anxiety**: An imbalanced gut can worsen these symptoms by disrupting the production of neurotransmitters like serotonin and GABA, which are important for mood regulation.
- **Cognitive changes**: "Brain fog" and memory issues during menopause may be linked to gut health, as the gut produces many of the body's neurotransmitters.

Inflammation and Menopause

Menopause often comes with increased levels of inflammation, partly due to hormonal changes. An unhealthy gut can worsen this inflammation, contributing to joint pain, fatigue, and mood disorders.

How to Support Gut-Brain Health During Menopause

To manage menopause symptoms and support the gut-brain connection:

- **Dietary Changes**: Focus on prebiotic and probiotic foods (e.g., yogurt, kefir, garlic, onions) to support a healthy gut microbiome.
- **Anti-inflammatory foods**: Include foods rich in omega-3 fatty acids, antioxidants, and fiber.
- **Stress Reduction**: Practices like yoga, meditation, and mindfulness can calm the gut-brain axis.
- **Probiotics**: Specific probiotic strains, such as *Lactobacillus* and *Bifidobacterium*, may help balance the microbiome and reduce inflammation.
- **Hormone Replacement Therapy (HRT)**: For some women, HRT may help restore balance in the gut and reduce menopausal symptoms.

The gut-brain connection is deeply intertwined with menopause. Hormonal changes during this time can disrupt gut health, which in turn influences mood, cognition, and inflammation. Supporting gut health through diet, lifestyle, and, if needed, medical interventions can help manage menopause symptoms.

GASTROINTESTINAL DISORDERS

Irritable Bowel Syndrome (IBS):

IBS affects about 10-25% of people in the U.S. and often feels like an ongoing battle in your stomach, with symptoms like pain, bloating, and irregular bowel movements. It's a complicated condition partly caused by dysbiosis. Changes in the gut-brain axis can disrupt how the gut works, affecting movement, gut lining, and bacteria balance. Since IBS is also linked to mental health conditions like anxiety and depression, it is extremely important to address physical and emotional health to manage symptoms effectively.

Inflammatory Bowel Disease (IBD):

Conditions like Crohn's disease and ulcerative colitis involve chronic inflammation in the digestive tract. This happens when the immune system goes into overdrive, attacking not just harmful invaders but also healthy tissues in the gut. The result is severe pain, diarrhea, and extreme fatigue, which can make daily life challenging. Gut bacteria imbalances can trigger this immune response, leading to ongoing inflammation. Making dietary changes and including probiotics can help restore balance and manage symptoms, offering relief for those living with IBD.

Celiac Disease:

Celiac disease happens when the immune system reacts to gluten, a protein found in wheat, barley, and rye. This reaction damages the small intestine, leading to symptoms like stomach pain, diarrhea, and difficulty absorbing nutrients. Gluten also makes the gut lining more "leaky," allowing harmful substances to enter the bloodstream and worsen inflammation. Managing celiac disease requires a strict gluten-free diet, which helps reduce symptoms and repair the gut lining.

Small Intestinal Bacterial Overgrowth (SIBO):

In SIBO, too many bacteria grow in the small intestine, leading to bloating, stomach pain, and poor nutrient absorption. To treat SIBO, you need to rebalance the gut bacteria with dietary changes, probiotics, and sometimes antibiotics to reduce the overgrowth.

METABOLIC AND ENDOCRINE DISORDERS

When people think about weight gain, they often think of extra calories or lack of exercise. But gut bacteria play a role, too. The composition of microbes in your gut can significantly influence how your body handles food, affecting metabolism and appetite. An imbalance in these bacteria can lead to increased fat storage and weight gain, contributing to obesity.

When it comes to Type 2 Diabetes, a condition where the body's ability to use insulin effectively is compromised, gut bacteria are also at play. Changes in these microbes can lead to insulin resistance, a precursor to diabetes. They can also trigger low-grade inflammation, further complicating the body's ability to manage blood sugar levels.

Non-Alcoholic Fatty Liver Disease (NAFLD) is also closely linked to gut health. Substances made by gut bacteria, called endotoxins, can travel to the liver and cause inflammation. This inflammation can lead to fat building up in the liver, which affects how well it works. Taking care of your gut through healthy eating, probiotics, and lifestyle changes is an important step in managing this condition. By understanding the gut's role in NAFLD, you can improve your liver health and other aspects of your overall well-being, like your metabolism and weight.

IMMUNE AND INFLAMMATORY CONDITIONS

The gut plays an important role in allergies and asthma. The development of gut bacteria early on is critical because it helps train your immune system to respond properly. If training doesn't go well, your immune system might mistakenly see things like pollen or dust as dangerous, triggering allergic reactions. Taking care of your gut health could help calm these immune responses and may reduce the severity of symptoms.

Psoriasis and eczema are also connected to gut health. These conditions are driven by inflammation, which can start in the gut and spread throughout the body. Your skin is a reflection of what's happening inside. When the stomach is inflamed, it can send signals that show up as rashes, itching, or irritation on the skin.

In psoriasis, the immune system speeds up the production of skin cells, creating scaly patches. The skin becomes itchy and inflamed with eczema, often due to the body's reaction to internal inflammation. Taking care of your gut can help reduce these inflammatory signals, calm the skin, and ease the discomfort caused by these conditions.

CARDIOVASCULAR DISEASES

Your gut sets the pace for your heart's health. Some gut bacteria produce substances like trimethylamine N-oxide (TMAO), which have been linked to a higher risk of heart disease. TMAO is made when gut bacteria break down certain nutrients found in red meat and eggs. It contributes to plaque buildup in your arteries, leading to atherosclerosis, a condition where the arteries harden and narrow. Imagine your arteries as highways and TMAO as the traffic jam that slows everything down, increasing your risk of heart attacks or strokes. Keeping your gut bacteria balanced through a healthy diet and lifestyle choices can help keep these "highways" clear and reduce the risk of blockages.

How Gut Health Affects Blood Pressure

High blood pressure, or hypertension, is also linked to your gut. When the balance of gut bacteria is disrupted, it can trigger inflammation that affects how your blood vessels work. Inflammation can make blood vessels tighten, which increases the pressure. This can lead to harmful substances being produced, further complicating things.

Taking care of your gut can lower inflammation and support healthy blood pressure levels. Eating fiber-rich foods, adding probiotics, and staying active are simple steps you can take to nurture your gut microbiome. These changes help reduce strain on your heart and promote better overall cardiovascular health.

CANCER

Colorectal cancer has been linked to gut health. When dysbiosis is present, it can lead to long-term inflammation. This creates an environment where tumors in the colon can form. The inflammation acts like fuel, helping cancer cells grow. Taking care of your gut through healthy habits can lower your risk of colorectal cancer. Eating more fiber-rich foods, staying physically active, and cutting back on red meat are ways to support a healthy gut and reduce this risk.

Gastric cancer involves Helicobacter pylori (H. pylori), a bacteria that settles in the stomach and can cause infections and inflammation. Over time, the damage from H. pylori and an imbalance in other gut bacteria can lead to changes in the stomach lining, turning healthy cells into cancerous ones. Along with early detection and treatment, you can also protect your stomach by eating healthy. Adding probiotics to help balance gut bacteria and avoiding excessive salt and processed foods are ways to protect yourself and keep your stomach healthy.

CHRONIC FATIGUE SYNDROME (CFS)

Chronic Fatigue Syndrome (CFS) causes an overwhelming lack of energy that even sleep can't fix. Research suggests that the gut might have something to do with this condition. When our systems become imbalanced, it can contribute to constant exhaustion. The gut affects inflammation and immune responses, which could also be key factors in this condition. By improving gut health, there's a chance one can reduce symptoms and regain energy.

KIDNEY DISEASE

Kidney disease may not seem like it's connected to the gut at first, but the two are in fact closely linked. Both the stomach and kidneys work to manage and remove toxins from the body. When the gut's bacteria are out of balance, it can lead to an overproduction of toxins that make the kidneys work harder. Taking care of your gut helps reduce the strain on your kidneys, potentially slowing the progression of kidney disease.

THYROID DISORDERS

Thyroid disorders, especially autoimmune conditions like Hashimoto's thyroiditis, also have ties to gut health. Since the gut plays a key role in regulating the immune system, when its balance is disrupted, it can trigger autoimmune responses. In Hashimoto's, the immune system mistakenly attacks the thyroid gland, which affects hormone production and metabolism. A healthy gut can help calm these immune responses, offering indirect support for thyroid health.

COMBATING INSOMNIA: GUT HEALTH FOR A GOOD NIGHT'S SLEEP

The balance of bacteria in your gut plays an important role in your sleep quality. Gut bacteria help produce melatonin, the hormone that regulates your sleep-wake cycle. A healthy gut will make enough melatonin to guide you into restful sleep. However, dysbiosis can disrupt your internal clock (circadian rhythm), making it harder to sleep. By taking care of your gut, you can improve your sleep patterns and wake up feeling rested and refreshed.

How Your Diet Affects Sleep and Gut Health

One way to improve sleep is by eating the right foods. For example:

- **Tryptophan-rich foods**: Tryptophan is an amino acid that helps your body make melatonin. Foods like turkey, chicken, seeds, and nuts are great sources and can help prepare your body for sleep when included in your evening meals.
- **Magnesium-rich foods**: Magnesium calms the nervous system and relaxes your muscles, promoting better sleep.

You can find magnesium in green leafy vegetables, almonds, and whole grains.
- **Limit caffeine and alcohol**: These can disrupt your sleep, so it's best to cut back on them, especially in the evening.

Probiotics and Prebiotics for Better Sleep

Probiotics and prebiotics can also help improve sleep by supporting gut health.

- **Probiotics**: Certain probiotic strains, like **Lactobacillus** and **Bifidobacterium**, may help improve sleep quality by influencing the production of neurotransmitters that regulate sleep. You will find these in yogurt, kefir, and miso, among others.
- **Prebiotics**: Be extra generous in using foods like garlic, onions, or anything of the prebiotic foods previously listedbto feed the good bacteria in your gut.This balance can help regulate your sleep cycle, making it easier to fall asleep and stay asleep.

Creating a Sleep-Friendly Routine

Along with diet, having a bedtime routine can make a big difference. Try these tips:

- **Dim the lights**: Lowering light levels signals your body that it's time to wind down.
- **Avoid screens**: Reduce screen time before bed, as the blue light from devices can interfere with melatonin production.
- **Relaxing activities**: Do calming activities like reading or gentle stretching to help your body relax.

- **Eat light meals**: Avoid heavy, hard-to-digest meals at night, and eat mindfully to prevent discomfort that could disrupt your sleep.

The Gut-Sleep Connection

By understanding how gut health affects sleep, you can begin to make changes so that you enjoy more restful nights and a more balanced life.

LEAKY GUT AND BAD METABOLITES - THEIR INFLUENCE ON DISEASE

Leaky Gut Syndrome describes a weakened gut lining. Imagine your gut lining as a tightly woven net that lets in nutrients while keeping harmful substances out. When this net gets holes, things like toxins and bacteria can leak into your bloodstream. This leakage triggers your immune system and causes inflammation, which can lead to other health problems, including autoimmune diseases. Many scientists agree that keeping your gut lining healthy is important for overall well-being.

The gut produces various substances, called metabolites, that can affect your health. Some of these, like short-chain fatty acids (SCFAs), are helpful. SCFAs support your immune system and reduce inflammation, promoting better health. But not all metabolites are good. For example, trimethylamine N-oxide (TMAO), linked to heart disease, shows how an imbalanced gut can produce harmful substances. This balance between helpful and detrimental metabolites shows us how important it is to maintain a healthy gut to encourage the production of beneficial compounds while minimizing harmful ones.

RECOGNIZING SIGNS OF GUT-RELATED ISSUES

Your body works like a finely tuned instrument, performing at its best when everything is in balance. But what happens when something feels off? Paying attention to the signs that your gut might be out of balance is the first step to fixing the problem. For example, if you're dealing with unexpected skin breakouts or constant bloating, these are clues from your gut signaling that something needs attention. Recognizing signs early can help you address imbalances and prevent bigger health issues in the future.

PHYSICAL SYMPTOMS OF GUT IMBALANCE

- **Brain Fog**:
    - Difficulty concentrating.
    - Feeling mentally slow or sluggish.
    - Trouble retaining information or staying on task.

- **Mood Swings and Emotional Imbalance**:
  - Increased feelings of anxiety or stress.
  - Irritability or snapping at others.
  - Sudden shifts from calm to anxious or down.
- **Sleep Problems**:
  - Difficulty falling asleep or staying asleep.
  - Frequent waking during the night.
  - Feeling tired and unrefreshed in the morning.
- **Hormonal Issues**:
  - Irregular menstrual cycles.
  - Energy highs and crashes throughout the day.
  - Difficulty maintaining emotional or mental stability.
- **Skin Issues**:
  - Unexpected breakouts or rashes.
  - Dry or irritated skin that doesn't respond to treatments.
- **Digestive Problems**:
  - Persistent bloating or gas.
  - Constipation or diarrhea.
  - Stomach pain or discomfort.

MENTAL SYMPTOMS OF GUT DISTRESS

- **Cognitive Issues (Brain Fog)**:
  - Sluggish, slow-thinking.
  - Difficulty concentrating or staying on task.
  - Trouble retaining information or processing thoughts.
  - Feeling like your brain is "stuck in molasses."
- **Emotional Instability**:
  - Increased feelings of anxiety or stress.
  - Sudden mood swings, from calm to anxious or upset.

- Unexplained irritability or snapping at loved ones.
- Feelings of sadness or being emotionally off-balance.
- **Sleep Disturbances**:
  - Trouble falling asleep or staying asleep.
  - Waking up frequently during the night.
  - Feeling drained or fatigued even after sleeping.
  - Restless sleep is tied to disrupted melatonin production.
- **Energy Fluctuations**:
  - Energy highs and lows throughout the day.
  - Feeling exhausted one moment and overly wired the next.
  - Difficulty maintaining steady energy levels.
- **Mood-Related Hormonal Issues**:
  - Fluctuations in serotonin levels affect mood regulation.
  - Difficulty staying calm or maintaining emotional clarity.

WHEN TO SEEK PROFESSIONAL HELP

Sometimes, gut discomfort requires more than dietary changes. Knowing when to get professional help is the only way to avoid serious health problems. Here are some signs that you should call a healthcare provider:

- **Severe abdominal pain**: If it feels sharp, like a twisting knife, don't ignore it.
- **Blood in your stool**: This could be a sign of an infection, inflammation, or another serious condition.
- **Persistent diarrhea**: Ongoing diarrhea that leaves you dehydrated and exhausted should be checked out.

WHO CAN HELP WITH GUT PROBLEMS?

- **Gastroenterologists**: These are specialists in digestive health and the best people to see for ongoing gut issues. They can diagnose and treat specific problems.
- **Nutritionists**: If your gut issues might be related to your diet, a nutritionist can assess your eating habits and suggest changes to help you feel better.

These professionals often work together to address your gut health from all angles, ensuring you get a complete care plan.

WHAT TO EXPECT AT YOUR APPOINTMENT

- **Health history**: Your doctor will ask about your symptoms, diet, lifestyle, and any family history of digestive issues.
- **Diagnostic tests**: Tests like:
  - **Endoscopy** (to view your digestive tract).
  - **Stool analysis** (to check your gut bacteria).
  - These tests help identify the exact cause of your symptoms.

TREATMENT OPTIONS

After diagnosis, your doctor may recommend a combination of treatments tailored to your needs:

- **Medications**: To reduce inflammation, fight infections, or manage symptoms.
- **Dietary changes**: Focus on foods that support gut healing and avoid irritants.

- **Probiotics or prebiotics**: To restore balance to your gut bacteria.
- **Stress management**: Techniques like yoga, meditation or a brisk walk can reduce gut-related symptoms. (insert at the end of chapter)
- **Elimination diets**: To identify and avoid food triggers.

SELF-ASSESSMENT TOOLS FOR EARLY DETECTION

Understanding your gut health means paying attention, as each symptom offers a clue about what's happening inside your body. A great way to start is by keeping a food and symptom diary. Simply write down what you eat and how you feel afterward—whether it's discomfort, bloating, or irregular digestion. Over time, you may notice patterns that reveal which foods work well for your gut and which ones don't. Online gut health questionnaires are also helpful. These ask questions about your diet, lifestyle, and symptoms to give you a snapshot of your gut's current state and point out areas needing attention.

Paying attention to your body's signals is just as important. Mindful eating can help you tune into how food affects you. This means noticing how your body responds to different meals. You can also take a few moments each day to check in with yourself, noting any physical or emotional changes. This daily habit helps you pick up on subtle signs your body might be giving off, allowing you to address potential issues early.

For those who enjoy a more hands-on approach, simple at-home tests can provide additional insights. For example, using saliva or urine strips to check your body's pH balance can provide clues about your digestion. Paying attention to changes in your bowel movements, such as their frequency, consistency, and color, can also offer valuable information about your gut health. However, these tests are not a replacement for professional diagnosis; they simply give you a glimpse of what's happening.

As you continue this journey, exploring practices like detoxification can further enhance both your gut health and overall well-being.

DETOXIFYING GUT AND MIND

Think of your body as a busy city where everything works together to keep things running smoothly. Just like this city needs regular clean-ups, your body needs to get rid of waste to keep it functioning well. When it comes to detoxifying your gut, there's a lot of misinformation out there that can lead to harmful practices. Detoxing isn't about extreme cleanses or miracle solutions; it's about helping your body do what it already does naturally.

Your body has its own detox system, and listening to it is essential. Overloading it with harsh detox programs can leave you feeling tired, lacking essential nutrients, or can even cause more digestive problems. The key is to work with your body, not against it, to help it stay healthy and balanced.

Gentle detox practices are a great way to cleanse without causing harm. Start by incorporating fiber-rich foods into your diet. They help move waste along the digestive tract and keep things regular. Fruits, vegetables, legumes, and whole grains are excellent sources of fiber and also nurture the beneficial bacteria in your gut for a healthy microbiome. Adding herbal teas like dandelion and peppermint can further enhance this process. Dandelion tea acts as a mild diuretic, helping flush out toxins, while peppermint tea soothes the digestive system, reducing bloating and discomfort.

Fasting has become a popular way to detox, and when done correctly, it can offer many benefits. Intermittent fasting, in particular, helps your gut rest and recover, which can improve digestion and even support weight loss. It involves alternating between eating and fasting periods, allowing your body time to reset its natural processes. A study from Arizona State University found that participants following an intermittent fasting and protein-pacing regimen experienced better gut health and weight loss compared to those on simple calorie restriction.

If you're new to fasting, start with shorter periods, like 12 to 16 hours, and gradually extend the time as your body gets used to it. Remember, fasting isn't about starving yourself—it's about giving your body a break from constant digestion so it can focus on repair and balance.

It's also worth noting that while intermittent fasting has potential benefits, it may not be suitable for everyone. Certain individuals with specific health conditions, pregnant women, or those with a history of eating disorders should exercise caution and seek medical advice before fasting.

Natural detox agents like activated charcoal and bentonite clay can also be beneficial. Activated charcoal binds to toxins in the digestive tract, preventing their absorption and aiding in their elimination. It's like a sponge that soaks up impurities, leaving your system cleaner. Bentonite clay works similarly, removing impurities and supporting gut health. However, these substances should be used sparingly and with caution. Overuse can lead to nutrient deficiencies, as they might also bind to essential vitamins and minerals. Always follow the recommended dosages and consult a healthcare professional if you're unsure.

Daily Detox Checklist

Create a personalized detox checklist to incorporate gentle detox practices into your routine. Include items like "Add a serving of leafy greens," "Enjoy a cup of herbal tea," and "Practice intermittent fasting for 14 hours." Use this checklist to track your progress and note any changes in how you feel over time. Remember, detoxification is a journey, and small, consistent steps lead to lasting results.

THE ROLE OF HYDRATION IN CLEANSING

Water is an essential part of your body's detox process, quietly working to keep you healthy. Staying hydrated is important because it helps remove toxins and waste that your body naturally produces. Think of water as your body's delivery and cleanup service, carrying nutrients to where they're needed and taking harmful substances away.

But water does more than just keep things moving. It also keeps your cells healthy. Every cell in your body needs water to work properly. Without water, cells can't do their jobs well. Water helps keep the outer layer of cells flexible, improves the absorption of nutrients, and supports the repair and growth of new cells.

To get enough water, start by checking your daily intake. While the standard "eight glasses a day" is a good guideline, your needs might vary depending on how active you are, the climate you live in, and your overall health. If you're more active or sweat a lot, you'll need extra water to stay hydrated. A simple way to tell if you're drinking enough is to check your urine—it should be a light yellow color.

You can also hydrate through food. Snacks like cucumbers and watermelon are packed with water, vitamins, and minerals. These hydrating foods can easily fit into your meals, whether in salads, smoothies, or as snacks.

To make drinking water more enjoyable, try adding natural flavors. Infused water is a simple and healthy way to stay hydrated. Add slices of lemon and mint to your water for a refreshing twist. Lemon gives you a boost of vitamin C, and mint helps with digestion. You can also experiment with other herbs like basil or fruits like strawberries to mix things up. Infused water adds flavor and nutrients without any added sugars or artificial ingredients.

Example: The Benefits of Lemons

Lemons offer a plethora of health benefits. From enhancing immunity to aiding digestion, lemons are versatile and delicious.

Immune Boosting Properties: Lemons are packed with vitamin C, a powerful antioxidant known for its immune-boosting properties. Regular consumption of lemon juice can help strengthen the body's defense against infections and illnesses.

Digestive Aid: The acidity of lemons can stimulate the production of digestive juices, promoting healthy digestion and alleviating symptoms of indigestion and bloating. A warm glass of lemon water in the morning can kickstart your digestive system.

Hydration Support: Lemon water provides a refreshing and flavorful way to meet your daily fluid intake goals. Adding a slice of lemon to your water not only enhances its taste but also encourages you to drink more water throughout the day.

Skin Rejuvenation: The vitamin C in lemons plays a crucial role in collagen synthesis, which is essential for maintaining healthy and youthful-looking skin. *Tip:* Applying lemon juice topically can help lighten dark spots, reduce acne, and brighten the complexion.

Detoxification: Lemons act as a natural detoxifier, helping to flush out toxins from the body and support liver function.

Weight Management: The soluble pectin fiber found in lemons helps curb cravings and promote feelings of fullness, making it easier to stick to a healthy eating plan.

Mood Enhancement: Lemons have been shown to have mood-boosting properties, helping to reduce stress and anxiety levels. Simply inhaling the aroma of lemon essential oil or sipping lemon tea can uplift your spirits and promote relaxation.

When your body doesn't have enough water, it can slow down digestion, making you feel uncomfortable and affecting how your body eliminates waste. Signs of dehydration include a dry mouth, headaches, low energy, and even dizziness or confusion in severe cases.

To prevent dehydration, drink water consistently throughout the day rather than all at once. Try carrying a water bottle and listening to your body to avoid dehydration and keep your body functioning at its best.

MENTAL DETOX TECHNIQUES FOR CLARITY

Sometimes, our minds can get cluttered with too many thoughts, worries, and distractions. A mental detox can help eliminate unnecessary clutter, reduce stress, make room for positive thinking, and create a calm mental space. This clarity can improve focus, balance your emotions, and help you handle challenges with greater ease.

Practices like mindfulness and meditation are excellent ways to clear your mind. They work like a reset button, letting you step away from daily chaos and find calm in the present moment. Guided visualization exercises can help transport you to peaceful places, like quiet beaches or calming forests, offering a mental escape from life's busyness. Mindful breathing is another simple way to feel calm—focusing on each breath helps you stay present, letting go of stress and creating a stronger connection between your mind and body.

Taking a break from screens is also a great way to mentally detox. Constant notifications and endless scrolling can overwhelm your mind. Setting boundaries, like limiting screen time or creating tech-free zones, can help you regain control. Try having a screen-free hour before bed to unwind or spend time reading, drawing, or walking instead.

Journaling can also help detox your mind. Writing things down that you're grateful for helps shift your focus toward positive thoughts. Reflective journaling can also help you process emotions and understand your thoughts. Try answering questions like, "What's one thing I accomplished today?" or "How can I approach tomorrow with a fresh perspective?" Writing gives you space to explore your feelings, leading to greater self-awareness and personal growth.

Mental detox doesn't happen all at once, but with small, consistent steps, you can create more clarity, balance, and peace in your life.

Mindfulness Wheel

Create a mindfulness wheel that includes different techniques like guided visualization, mindful breathing, and tech-free activities. Use this wheel as a visual guide to select a daily practice. This can help you incorporate various methods into your life.

INTEGRATING DETOX INTO A DAILY ROUTINE

Regular detoxification helps your body eliminate accumulated toxins, supports your immune system, and reduces the risk of chronic illnesses. It's a form of preventative health care that leads to improved energy levels, clearer skin, and better digestion.

Try sipping warm lemon water to kickstart your digestive system and practicing daily meditation to calm your mind. This can also help reduce cortisol levels, which can be beneficial for your gut health. Even just five minutes of focused breathing or mindful reflection can make a noticeable difference in your day.

Nutrition is extremely important for detoxification. By choosing to eat a rainbow of fruits and vegetables, you can provide your body with a variety of nutrients and antioxidants that aid in the detox process. Each color represents different phytonutrients, all working together to support your body's natural cleansing mechanisms. Opting for whole foods over processed options is another great choice. Whole foods are less likely to contain preservatives and additives that can burden your body's detox pathways. Think of each meal as an opportunity to nourish your body, choosing ingredients that are as close to their natural state as possible.

Use simple strategies to help you stay on track. Set reminders for hydration breaks throughout the day, and consider using apps to remind you to take a sip of water or stand up and stretch. Stock your pantry with healthy foods, like nuts, seeds, and whole grains, and keep a variety of fresh fruits and vegetables on hand. This makes it easier to prepare wholesome meals and snacks, reducing the temptation to reach for less healthy options.

With time and consistency, these small steps can lead to powerful health benefits, supporting not just your physical well-being but also your mental clarity and emotional balance.

LIFESTYLE CHANGES FOR GUT-BRAIN HARMONY

Exercise, in particular, can improve your gut microbiome. Beyond burning calories or building muscle, regular physical activity creates an environment where beneficial bacteria flourish, digestion runs smoothly, and mental health is improved.

BOOSTING GUT HEALTH THROUGH MOVEMENT

Regular physical activity plays a vital role in keeping your gut microbiome healthy and balanced. As this ecosystem helps break down food, absorb nutrients, and protect you from harmful bacteria, exercise boosts the number of "good" microbes, making the microbiome more diverse.

Exercise also helps your digestion by keeping things moving smoothly. Physical activity stimulates the muscles in your intestines, which allows food to move more efficiently through your digestive system. This can prevent constipation, support nutrient absorption, and create a healthier gut environment.

Not all types of exercise affect gut health in the same way. Aerobic exercises like walking, cycling, and swimming are especially good for the gut. They raise your heart rate, improve circulation, and encourage the growth of healthy gut bacteria. Aerobic activities also release endorphins, which improve your mood and reduce feelings of stress, anxiety, and depression. Strength training also supports gut health by building muscle and enhancing metabolism, which helps your body manage glucose (blood sugar) and fat better.

When starting an exercise routine, begin with activities you enjoy and slowly increase how long or how hard you exercise. For example, you could take walks on some days and do strength training on others. Aim for at least 30 minutes of moderate exercise most days of the week. Even small amounts of consistent movement can have a significant impact on your health.

Make other changes like taking the stairs instead of the elevator, parking farther away to walk more, or having walking meetings at work. You can also make exercise more fun by doing it with others. Join a fitness class, invite friends for a hike, or play a team sport.

Exercise also supports your mind. It increases blood flow to the brain and helps regulate stress by balancing the body's HPA axis (which manages your stress response). This can improve mood, lower anxiety, and boost self-esteem. Exercise gives you a sense of achievement and acts as a healthy distraction from negative thoughts.

Exercise Journal

To make exercise a consistent part of your life:

1. Consider keeping an exercise journal.
2. Track your workouts, noting the type, duration, and intensity of each session.
3. Reflect on how you feel before and after exercising, both physically and mentally.

This holds you accountable and helps you identify patterns and preferences. Over time, you may discover which activities bring you the most joy and benefit, guiding you toward a personalized exercise routine that supports your gut-brain harmony.

TOOLS FOR EMOTIONAL BALANCE

Finding emotional balance can be difficult. Life often pulls you in many directions, leaving your mind overwhelmed and in need of a break. Mindfulness and relaxation techniques can help you find this calm while also improving your gut health.

Try guided imagery, where you close your eyes and imagine peaceful, relaxing scenes—like sitting on a quiet beach or walking through a forest. This simple practice can lower stress and anxiety, triggering your body's natural relaxation response. A study published in *Psychoneuroendocrinology* found that mindfulness-based stress reduction (MBSR) is associated with a more diverse and balanced gut microbiome, which is linked to better gut health.

Other complementary therapies can also help. For example, aromatherapy uses essential oils to calm your emotions. When you smell certain oils or apply them to your skin, they affect a part of the brain called the limbic system, which controls your mood. This helps lower stress, which is good news for your gut health since stress can disrupt digestion. Essential oils like lavender, peppermint, and chamomile have calming effects. Research in the *Journal of Pharmaceutical Health Care and Sciences* confirmed that aromatherapy can influence the immune and autonomic nervous systems.

Another helpful practice is acupuncture, which works by inserting tiny needles into specific points on your body to help balance your energy. A study in the *Journal of Acupuncture and Meridian Studies* reported that acupuncture can reduce stress by releasing endorphins (your body's "feel-good" chemicals) and lowering cortisol, the stress hormone.

Adding self-care habits to your day can also help you feel more emotionally balanced. Journaling is a great way to start. Write down your thoughts and feelings each day to reflect and release emotions you may not even realize are weighing you down. Practicing gratitude is another good habit to add to your routine. Each day, try writing down three things you're thankful for. Focusing on the good things in your life helps you feel calmer and more content, which benefits your overall well-being.

These practices help you manage stress and take care of both your mind and gut. However, you can't completely remove stress from your life; you can only learn to handle it in healthier ways. The important thing is to find something that works for you.

MANAGING STRESS FOR GUT-BRAIN HEALTH

Life has its way of throwing curveballs. From daily commutes to meeting deadlines, stress can be constant. As we've already established, your body's response to stress isn't just in your mind but in your gut, too. This amazing gut-brain connection is a balance between your mental state and digestive health. When stress hits, this balance can wobble. Understanding how your body processes stress is key to regaining control over both your mind and gut.

UNDERSTANDING STRESS

Your body has a built-in alarm system called the stress response system, which works like a fire alarm, ready to activate when it detects a threat. At the center of this system is the hypothalamic-pituitary-adrenal (HPA) axis—a communication pathway that connects your brain to your adrenal glands. When you experience stress, your brain sends a signal to the HPA axis, triggering the release of stress hormones like adrenaline and cortisol. These hormones prepare your body to respond quickly: your heart rate increases, your focus sharpens, and your body enters "fight or flight" mode. While this is helpful in avoiding danger or meeting a deadline, long-term stress can seriously harm your health, including your gut.

Acute Stress vs. Chronic Stress

Acute stress comes suddenly but doesn't stick around for long. For example, feeling nervous before a presentation or startled by loud noise. Once the stress passes, your body returns to normal. You might feel a little shaky but relieved.

Chronic stress, on the other hand, is like a constant drizzle that never stops. This type of stress lasts for long periods and often comes from things like ongoing work pressure, financial worries, or personal struggles. Over time, the constant release of stress hormones wears your body down, increasing your risk for anxiety, depression, and digestive disorders. A 2021 study published in *Neurobiology of Stress* also confirmed that chronic stress can disrupt the gut-brain axis, impacting both mental health and gut function.

How Stress Affects Your Gut

When you're stressed, your gut often reacts in ways you might not expect. Stress increases gut permeability, which means your gut lining becomes more porous. This condition is usually called a "leaky gut," where undigested food particles and toxins leak into your bloodstream. Your immune system sees these as threats, which can trigger inflammation and discomfort. A study published in *Frontiers in Microbiology* found that stress can alter gut permeability, increasing the risk of inflammation and immune responses.

Stress also impacts the balance of bacteria in your gut, known as your gut microbiome. This bacteria helps with digestion, immunity, and even mood regulation. When stress disrupts this balance, you might experience bloating, irregular bowel movements, and stomach pain. Research in *Brain, Behavior, and Immunity* shows that stress reduces the diversity of gut bacteria, which can worsen digestive issues.

Psychosomatic Symptoms: How Stress Feels in the Gut

Stress doesn't just harm the gut; it can also cause physical symptoms. These are called psychosomatic symptoms. It's like having a "knot in your stomach" before a big event. That's the gut responding to stress signals. Stress can also change your appetite—you might overeat comfort foods to cope or lose your appetite altogether. Digestive problems like abdominal pain, bloating, or nausea without a clear medical cause are often linked to stress.

Reflect and Understand

Think about a recent time when stress affected your digestion or appetite. Did you experience bloating, pain, or changes in your hunger? Write down how it made you feel and when it happened. Understanding your body's stress response helps you recognize the connection between your emotions and your gut health. By noticing these patterns, you can take steps to manage stress more effectively.

CORTISOL'S IMPACT ON GUT HEALTH

Cortisol, the "stress hormone," is produced by your adrenal glands and plays a huge role in keeping your body functioning. In short bursts, cortisol is helpful—it gives you the boost you need to handle challenges or unexpected situations. However, when cortisol levels stay high for too long, it can negatively affect your body, especially your gut.

How Cortisol Impacts Digestion

When you're under constant stress, your body stays in "fight-or-flight" mode, meaning it focuses all its energy on handling the perceived threat. This takes energy away from digestion, slowing it down. As a result, you may experience bloating, constipation, or an unsettled stomach. A 2019 study published in *Psychoneuroendocrinology* found that elevated cortisol levels are associated with slower digestion and increased gastrointestinal symptoms like abdominal pain.

Cortisol and Gut Bacteria Imbalance

Cortisol also disrupts the microbiome, where trillions of good and bad microorganisms help with digestion, immunity, and even mood regulation. Prolonged stress and high cortisol levels can reduce the number of beneficial bacteria, allowing harmful bacteria to thrive. This imbalance can lead to digestive problems and even weaken your immune system.

Cortisol and "Leaky Gut"

Another effect of elevated cortisol is something we've already mentioned: the breakdown of the gut lining, a condition known as increased gut permeability or "leaky gut." The gut lining allows nutrients to pass through while keeping harmful substances out; when cortisol weakens this structure, it creates tiny gaps that let toxins, undigested food particles, and bacteria leak into the bloodstream. This can trigger inflammation and cause fatigue, joint pain, and autoimmune conditions. A 2020 study in *Nutrients* confirmed that prolonged stress and cortisol exposure contribute to gut permeability, inflammation, and related systemic health problems.

How to Lower Cortisol and Protect Gut Health

Managing your cortisol levels is essential for your gut and overall health. One of the best ways to do this is through regular physical activity. As previously mentioned, exercise is a natural stress reliever that reduces cortisol while improving mood and energy levels. Walking, dancing, swimming, or yoga can help bring your body and mind back to balance. A 2019 study published in *The Journal of Sports Science & Medicine* found that regular exercise significantly reduced cortisol levels and improved gut health markers.

Relaxation techniques like meditation, deep breathing, and mindfulness also help activate your body's relaxation response, calming your nervous system and decreasing stress hormones. This is backed up by a 2021 study in *Psychosomatic Medicine*, which found that mindfulness-based techniques reduced cortisol and improved symptoms of stress-related digestive issues.

Understanding how cortisol affects your body allows you to take steps to manage stress and protect your gut health. By incorporating regular exercise and relaxation techniques into your daily routine, you can support a healthier gut and improve your overall well-being.

STRESS REDUCTION MINDFULNESS PRACTICES

Mindfulness meditation is a simple way to manage stress. It begins with focused breathing exercises, which calm your mind, slow your heart rate, and ease tension.

To start, find a quiet, comfortable space. Sit or lie down in a position that feels good. Close your eyes and focus on your breathing:

Deep Breathing Exercise:

- Inhale slowly and deeply through your nose for 4 seconds.
- Hold your breath for 4 seconds.
- Exhale slowly through your mouth for 6 seconds.
- Repeat this process for 5-10 minutes.

This simple breathing method activates the parasympathetic nervous system, helping your body relax and reduce stress hormones. Studies support that deep breathing exercises significantly reduce cortisol levels.

Another great mindfulness practice is the body scan technique, which helps you tune into areas of tension in your body and consciously release them.

Body Scan Exercise:

- Lie down or sit comfortably and close your eyes.
- Start at the top of your head and mentally "scan" down your body, paying attention to how each area feels.
- Pause on any areas of tension (like your shoulders, neck, or stomach) and take a deep breath in. As you exhale, imagine the stress melting away.
- Move down your body slowly until you reach your toes.

The body scan makes you aware of the stress you hold in your muscles and helps you release it. Body scans have been proven to improve symptoms of stress and sleep quality in adults experiencing anxiety.

The Science Behind Mindfulness and Stress Reduction

Research supports the benefits of mindfulness meditation for stress and gut health. Mindfulness helps reduce cortisol levels, which can harm your digestion and immune function. A 2016 study published in *Biological Psychiatry* found that individuals who practiced mindfulness meditation for 8 weeks experienced a significant reduction in cortisol and improved emotional resilience.

Mindfulness can also positively impact gut health. Chronic stress disrupts the gut microbiome by reducing beneficial bacteria and increasing harmful microbes. Regular mindfulness helps regulate the gut-brain axis, improving gut microbial diversity, which is essential for digestion and immunity.

Bringing Mindfulness into Your Life

Today, finding time for anything extra might feel difficult, but the good news is that even a few minutes each day can make a big difference.

Here are simple tips to make mindfulness a habit:

- Start your morning with 5 minutes of deep breathing or a body scan to set a calm tone for the day.
- During the day, take short "mindful breaks." Pause, close your eyes, and focus on your breathing for a minute.
- In the evening, try progressive relaxation—start at your feet, tense each muscle group briefly, and then relax it completely. This technique prepares your body for restful sleep.

Over time, mindfulness will feel natural, helping you manage stress, improve digestion, and restore balance to your life.

QUICK STRESS-REDUCTION TECHNIQUES

Sometimes, stress hits when you least expect it. You're in the middle of a meeting, stuck in traffic, or perhaps juggling tasks at home. These moments call for rapid stress-relief techniques. Some of these methods have already been mentioned but it seemed necessary to relist them here.

Quick and effective stress relief techniques you can use anywhere to calm your mind and body:

Deep Breathing (4-7-8 Technique)

- Inhale through your nose for 4 seconds.
- Hold your breath for 7 seconds.
- Exhale slowly through your mouth for 8 seconds.
- Repeat for 4-5 cycles.
- *This simple technique can slow your heart rate and reduce anxiety quickly.*

Box Breathing

- Inhale through your nose for 4 seconds.
- Hold your breath for 4 seconds.
- Exhale through your mouth for 4 seconds.
- Pause for 4 seconds before repeating.
- *Navy SEALs use this method to manage stress quickly and effectively.*

Grounding Exercise (5-4-3-2-1)

- Identify five things you can see.
- Acknowledge four things you can touch.
- Notice three things you can hear.
- Focus on two things you can smell.
- Recognize one thing you can taste.
- *This Technique helps bring you back to the present moment and reduce racing thoughts.*

Tense and Release (Progressive Muscle Relaxation)

- Tense a muscle group (like your fists or shoulders) for 5 seconds.
- Relax it entirely as you exhale.
- Move through different muscle groups: shoulders, arms, legs, and face.
- *This helps release built-up tension in your body quickly.*

Quick Walk or Movement Break

- Take a brisk 5-10 minute walk or stretch your body.
- Move your arms, roll your neck, or do light jumping jacks.
- *Physical movement releases endorphins, lowers cortisol, and clears your mind.*

Mindful Breathing

- Focus on your breath for 1 minute.
- Inhale deeply through your nose, exhale slowly through your mouth.
- Pay attention to the rise and fall of your chest or abdomen.
- *This anchors your mind, lowers stress, and brings calm quickly.*

Splash Cold Water on Your Face

- Splash your face with cold water or hold a cold compress to your cheeks.
- *This stimulates the vagus nerve, which can calm your nervous system immediately.*

Visualization

- Close your eyes and picture a peaceful scene—a beach, forest, or favorite memory.
- Breathe deeply as you imagine the sights, sounds, and smells.
- *Guided imagery can quickly shift your focus and reduce stress.*

Aromatherapy

- Keep a small bottle of calming essential oils like lavender, peppermint, or eucalyptus.
- Inhale deeply for a few seconds or apply a drop to your wrist.
- *Essential oils can have an immediate calming effect.*

Quick Gratitude Reflection

- Pause for 1 minute and think of 3 things you're grateful for right now.
- This can be simple: "I'm grateful for fresh air, my comfy chair, and my favorite song."
- *Shifting your mindset to positivity reduces stress and improves mood.*

Laughter Therapy

- Watch a funny video, listen to a joke, or think of something that made you laugh recently.
- *Laughter releases endorphins and relaxes your body.*

Power Pose

- Stand tall with your feet apart and your hands on your hips for 2 minutes (like a superhero pose).
- Breathe deeply while holding this posture.
- *Research shows this boosts confidence and reduces cortisol levels.*

Listen to Calming Music

- Play soothing music, nature sounds, or a favorite relaxing song for a few minutes.
- Focus on the melody and let it calm your mind.

Count Backward

- Slowly count backward from 20 to 1, focusing on each number.
- *This helps distract your mind and lower stress quickly.*

Sip Herbal Tea

- Take a few minutes to sip calming teas like chamomile, peppermint, or lemon balm.
- Focus on the warmth and aroma to help you feel grounded.

Chew Gum:

- A surprising stress reliever, chewing gum can reduce cortisol levels and improve focus.

SUPPORTING THE MICROBIOME AND ADAPTING YOUR JOURNEY FOR SUSTAINABILITY

Microbial diversity is essential for a healthy gut. One study published in *Nature* (2012) demonstrated that greater gut microbiome diversity correlates with lower risks of metabolic and autoimmune diseases. While another found that individuals with diverse microbiomes have improved nutrient absorption and metabolic function (Heiman & Greenway, 2016).

How Your Environment Shapes Your Microbiome: Urban vs. Rural Living

Your external environment affects your internal ecosystem. The microbes you encounter every day play an important role in shaping your gut microbiome.

Urban living exposes you to a limited range of microbes compared to rural areas. Pollution, processed foods, and a lack of natural environments can upset the balance of your gut bacteria. Research has shown that urban environments tend to be associated with lower microbial diversity in the gut, which is linked to higher rates of chronic diseases and mental health conditions.

According to *Environmental Health Perspectives* (2020), pollution adds another layer of complexity. Heavy metals, chemicals, and airborne particles can disrupt the microbiome and increase inflammation in the body. This imbalance doesn't just affect digestion, but it also contributes to conditions like anxiety and depression by altering the gut-brain axis.

The Rural Advantage

In contrast, rural areas offer a richer microbial environment. Exposure to soil, animals, and plants introduces a wider variety of beneficial microbes into the gut. Studies published in *Science* (2016) show that individuals living in rural settings have a more diverse microbiome, which is linked to stronger immunity and a lower risk of allergies and autoimmune conditions.

Hygiene: Finding the Right Balance

Cleanliness also impacts the microbiome. Over-sanitizing can strip away both harmful and beneficial bacteria, reducing microbial diversity. While hygiene is important, using harsh chemical cleaners can have negative consequences. Studies have shown that overuse of chemical disinfectants reduces beneficial microbes in the home, impacting the gut microbiome.

Try opting for natural cleaning products that are less disruptive to microbial communities. These allow beneficial bacteria to remain while still keeping things clean. Striking a balance between cleanliness and exposure to natural microbes can help build a more robust microbiome.

Connecting with Nature to Boost Your Microbiome

Spending time outdoors can introduce beneficial microbes to your system. Gardening, hiking, or simply walking in a park allows you to come into contact with soil and air filled with microbial life. Soil, in particular, contains bacteria like *Mycobacterium vaccae*, which has been shown to improve immune function and reduce inflammation (*Immunology*, 2019). The outdoors can enrich your microbiome, aiding digestion, boosting immunity, and supporting mental health.

Use Antibiotics with Care

Antibiotics, while lifesaving, can also disrupt the balance of the microbiome. Medications often eliminate harmful bacteria but also wipe out beneficial ones, leading to dysbiosis. A study in *Nature Communications* (2019) highlighted that a single course of antibiotics can significantly reduce gut microbial diversity, leaving the system vulnerable to infections and inflammation.

To mitigate this, consider taking probiotics during and after antibiotic treatment. Foods like yogurt, kefir, and fermented vegetables can also provide a natural boost to the recovery process.

THE IMPORTANCE OF TRACKING PROGRESS

Tracking your progress can be as simple as jotting down what you eat and how you feel. By recording your dietary intake and symptoms, you can identify patterns. Maybe you notice that stress at work often coincides with digestive discomfort or that certain foods trigger brain fog. This allows you to make informed decisions about what to eat and how to manage stress effectively. Apps are also super helpful and can track everything from meals to mood swings. Many even offer insights and suggestions based on your data.

Here are a few great options:

Cara Care: IBS, FODMAP Tracker

This app allows you to monitor food intake, stress levels, bowel movements, and abdominal discomfort, creating a personalized health diary to identify patterns and triggers.

Nerva

Utilizing gut-directed hypnotherapy, Nerva aims to alleviate IBS symptoms by addressing the gut-brain connection through hypnotherapy sessions, educational content, and breathing exercises.

mySymptoms Food Diary

This app enables you to log daily activities, including IBS symptoms, meals, exercise, and sleep quality, helping to identify correlations between lifestyle factors and digestive health.

Elsavie

Focused on gut health tracking, Elsavie assists in pinpointing the root causes of common IBS symptoms like constipation, bloating, and diarrhea, offering additional features such as stool, water, and supplement trackers.

Injoy: Gut Health Tracker

Injoy provides tools to monitor digestive health, offering personalized wellness plans with specific dietary, supplementary, and lifestyle recommendations based on individual data.

To better understand how your body is working, biomarkers can provide helpful insights. Biomarkers are measurable indicators that show what's happening inside your body. For example, tracking inflammation markers like C-reactive protein (CRP) can uncover hidden inflammation that might be influencing your mood or digestion. Stool tests, on the other hand, give a snapshot of your gut's microbiome. They show which types of bacteria are thriving and which are lacking. Although these tests aren't meant to diagnose specific conditions, they provide useful information about your gut health. Just remember, results can vary, so it's always a good idea to consult a healthcare professional if you have any concerns.

ADJUSTING DIETARY AND LIFESTYLE HABITS

Being flexible with your daily habits and going with the flow is important. When it comes to eating and exercising, being open to change is key. For instance, you might follow a meal plan that seemed ideal, only to realize it doesn't meet your body's current needs. Perhaps you need more fiber, or a different exercise routine feels better. Paying attention to these signals and adjusting your habits helps you stay on track with your health goals.

It's also important to spot habits that might be getting in your way. Maybe it's grabbing a late-night snack that affects your sleep or drinking too much caffeine. Even small patterns can hold you back from feeling your best. Pay attention to how certain foods and actions make you feel. Do they give you energy or leave you feeling tired? This awareness is the first step toward positive change. Once you identify what's not working, you can begin to replace those habits with ones that support your well-being.

Taking small, manageable steps is often more effective than overhauling your entire life. Start by adding one serving of vegetables to your meals each day to increase your fiber intake. Or, try simple changes like taking the stairs instead of the elevator to get more movement into your day. The idea is to make changes feel achievable so that you're motivated to keep going.

Creating and sticking to new habits is where lasting progress happens. Start with realistic goals that you can reach without too much stress. Give yourself some flexibility to adjust as needed.

PERSONALIZING YOUR GUT-BRAIN WELLNESS PLAN

Wellness is not a one-size-fits-all solution; it's unique to each person. Creating a personalized gut-brain wellness plan should fit your lifestyle, preferences, and needs. Everyone has different dietary and lifestyle requirements. By tailoring your nutrition and habits to what works best for you, your wellness journey becomes more enjoyable and sustainable.

Personalizing your nutrition plan is about ensuring you get the right balance of carbohydrates, proteins, and fats to match your energy needs and health goals. For example, if you need sustained energy throughout the day, focus on meals with balanced portions of macronutrients. Here's a list of macronutrients:

Carbohydrates

- Whole grains (e.g., oats, quinoa, brown rice)
- Legumes (e.g., lentils, chickpeas, black beans)
- Fruits (e.g., bananas, apples, berries)
- Vegetables (e.g., sweet potatoes, carrots, broccoli)
- High-fiber foods (e.g., chia seeds, flaxseeds)

Proteins

- Lean meats (e.g., chicken, turkey)
- Fish (e.g., salmon, tuna, mackerel)
- Plant-based proteins (e.g., tofu, tempeh, edamame)
- Eggs
- Dairy products (e.g., yogurt, cottage cheese)
- Protein-rich legumes (e.g., lentils, black beans)

Fats

- Healthy oils (e.g., olive oil, avocado oil)
- Nuts and seeds (e.g., almonds, walnuts, chia seeds)
- Fatty fish (e.g., salmon, sardines)
- Avocados
- Nut butters (e.g., almond butter, peanut butter)

Gut-Friendly Foods (Supporting Macronutrients)

- Probiotic-rich foods (e.g., yogurt, kimchi, sauerkraut)
- Prebiotic-rich foods (e.g., garlic, onions, asparagus)
- High-fiber vegetables (e.g., kale, spinach, artichokes)

When you include foods that are both nutritious and enjoyable, it's easier to stick with your plan long-term.

Exercise is another area where customization is important. Some people enjoy the intensity of a fast-paced workout, while others prefer calming activities like yoga or tai chi. The secret is to choose activities that you genuinely enjoy. If working out feels like a chore, keeping up with it is harder. The best workout is the one you love doing because consistency is what leads to actual results.

Stress management practices should also match your personality and interests. Not everyone enjoys traditional meditation, and that's okay. Explore alternatives like guided imagery, mindful movement, or yoga styles that resonate with your values or interests. You might also combine listening to music, painting, coloring, or journaling with relaxation techniques to make them more engaging. A personalized wellness plan is not about following someone else's formula—it's about designing a routine that works for you.

MAINTAINING MOTIVATION AND OVERCOMING SETBACKS

Staying motivated can be challenging. At first, you might feel excited, but that enthusiasm can fade when results don't show up quickly. It's easy to feel frustrated when your hard work doesn't pay off right away, making it tempting to give up. Boredom is another hurdle. When routines become repetitive, your efforts might feel like a chore instead of a choice.

However, there are several strategies to help you stay motivated. Set both short-term and long-term goals to keep yourself moving forward. Celebrate each small win with a reward—whether it's treating yourself to a favorite activity, a relaxing break, or even just recognizing your progress.

When setbacks happen, think of them as part of your growth story. Instead of feeling like you've failed, view these moments as opportunities to learn and adjust. Being flexible and open to change shows strength, not weakness. Remember, every setback can be a chance to come back stronger and more determined.

Self-reflection is another way to stay motivated. Take time to appreciate your progress, no matter how small it might seem.

Practicing gratitude for what you've achieved builds a sense of positivity and confidence. On tough days, be kind to yourself. Treat yourself with the same patience and encouragement you'd offer a close friend. Self-compassion fuels your resilience, making it easier to keep going.

CULTIVATING A GROWTH MINDSET FOR PERSONAL DEVELOPMENT

Imagine facing every challenge as a chance to grow. That's what having a growth mindset is all about. It's the belief that with effort and persistence, you can improve your abilities and overcome obstacles. In terms of health, this means understanding that struggles don't mean failure. Instead, they're lessons that help you adapt and move forward.

A growth mindset has many benefits, especially for personal development and health. It helps you bounce back from tough times with resilience, making it easier to keep going when things get complicated. When you believe that effort leads to progress, you're more motivated to take action and stay committed to your goals.

You can develop a growth mindset by changing the way you talk to yourself. Your thoughts influence how you see challenges, so practice shifting negative self-talk into positive affirmations. For example, replace "I can't do this" with "I'm still learning how to do this." Another key strategy is setting realistic and achievable goals. Break big goals into smaller steps that feel manageable. Each small accomplishment boosts your confidence and keeps you motivated to tackle the next challenge. This approach helps you stay focused without feeling overwhelmed.

Having a growth mindset does not mean in any way pretending challenges aren't difficult and oftentimes disheartening. Instead, it means understanding that difficulties are part of the journey. By adopting this mindset, you can take charge of your progress. As you reflect on these ideas, think about how applying them can create a strong foundation for improvement in all areas of your life.

RECIPES : SEVEN-DAY MEAL PLAN

Here's a collection of gut-brain wellness recipes for breakfast, lunch, dinner, and snacks. Each recipe includes ingredients that promote gut health and support the gut-brain connection with the three pillars- fiber-rich foods, fermented options, and omega-3s.

BREAKFAST RECIPES

Gut-Boosting Chia Pudding

Ingredients:

- Three tablespoons chia seeds
- One cup unsweetened almond milk (or other gut-friendly milk)
- One teaspoon of honey or maple syrup
- One tablespoon of ground flaxseeds

- ½ cup fresh berries (blueberries, raspberries, or strawberries)

Instructions:

1. Mix chia seeds, almond milk, and honey in a bowl or jar.
2. Let it sit for 10 minutes, stirring occasionally, until the seeds absorb the liquid and thicken.
3. Top with flaxseeds and fresh berries before serving.

Fermented Veggie Omelet

Ingredients:

- Two large eggs (or substitute with gut-friendly plant-based eggs)
- One tablespoon of kefir or Greek yogurt
- ½ cup spinach, chopped
- ¼ cup sauerkraut or kimchi (making instructions at the end of Recipes)
- One teaspoon of olive oil

Instructions:

1. Beat the eggs with kefir or Greek yogurt for extra probiotics.
2. Heat olive oil in a skillet over medium heat. Add spinach and sauté until wilted.
3. Pour the egg mixture into the skillet. Add sauerkraut or kimchi on top.
4. Cook until set, fold, and serve.

Avocado Toast with Fermented Veggies

Ingredients:

- One slice of whole-grain or sourdough bread
- ½ avocado, mashed
- ¼ cup sauerkraut or kimchi
- A pinch of sea salt and chili flakes

Instructions:

1. Toast the bread.
2. Spread mashed avocado and top with sauerkraut or kimchi. Sprinkle with sea salt and chili flakes.

Gut-Nurturing Smoothie Bowl

Ingredients:

- 1 cup unsweetened almond milk
- ½ banana (frozen)
- ½ cup spinach
- One tablespoon of chia seeds
- ½ cup granola (low sugar)

Instructions:

1. Blend almond milk, banana, spinach, and chia seeds until thick.
2. Pour into a bowl and top with granola.

Probiotic Yogurt Parfait

Ingredients:

- 1 cup plain Greek yogurt or dairy-free probiotic yogurt
- ½ cup granola
- ¼ cup fresh berries
- One tablespoon of hemp seeds

Instructions:

1. Layer yogurt, granola, and berries in a glass.
2. Sprinkle hemp seeds on top before serving.

Turmeric-Spiced Oats

Ingredients:

- ½ cup rolled oats
- 1 cup almond milk
- ½ teaspoon turmeric powder
- One tablespoon honey
- A pinch of cinnamon

Instructions:

1. Cook oats in almond milk with turmeric and cinnamon.
2. Sweeten with honey and serve warm.

Blueberry Buckwheat Pancakes

Ingredients:

- ½ cup buckwheat flour
- ½ cup almond milk
- One egg (or flax egg for vegan)
- ¼ cup blueberries
- One teaspoon of coconut oil for cooking

Instructions:

1. Mix flour, milk, and egg. Fold in blueberries.
2. Cook pancakes in coconut oil until golden.

LUNCH RECIPES

Gut-Healing Grain Bowl

Ingredients:

- 1 cup cooked quinoa
- ½ cup roasted sweet potatoes
- ¼ avocado, sliced
- ¼ cup fermented veggies (like kimchi or pickled carrots)
- One handful of arugula or baby spinach
- Two tablespoons of tahini dressing

Instructions:

1. Arrange quinoa, sweet potatoes, avocado, and arugula in a bowl.

2. Top with fermented veggies and drizzle with tahini dressing.

Omega-3 Salmon Salad

Ingredients:

- 1 cup mixed greens
- 3 ounces cooked salmon (rich in omega-3s)
- ½ cup roasted beets
- One tablespoon pumpkin seeds
- One tablespoon of olive oil
- Juice of ½ lemon

Instructions:

1. Toss mixed greens, roasted beets, and pumpkin seeds in a bowl.
2. Top with salmon.
3. Drizzle with olive oil and lemon juice before serving.

Miso Veggie Noodle Bowl

Ingredients:

- 1 cup cooked soba noodles
- One tablespoon of miso paste
- ½ cup steamed broccoli
- ½ cup shredded carrots
- One boiled egg (optional)

Instructions:

1. Dissolve miso paste in hot water to create broth.
2. Add noodles, veggies, and eggs. Serve warm.

Grain-Free Cauliflower Rice Bowl

Ingredients:

- 1 cup cauliflower rice
- ¼ cup chickpeas (roasted)
- ½ avocado, sliced
- One tablespoon of tahini dressing

Instructions:

1. Sauté cauliflower rice for 5 minutes.
2. Top with roasted chickpeas, avocado, and tahini.

Mediterranean Lentil Salad

Ingredients:

- 1 cup cooked lentils
- ½ cup diced cucumbers
- ¼ cup crumbled feta (optional)
- Two tablespoons of olive oil
- Juice of ½ lemon

Instructions:

1. Toss lentils, cucumbers, and feta in olive oil and lemon juice.

Collard Green Wraps

Ingredients:

- Two large collard green leaves
- ½ cup hummus
- ¼ cup shredded carrots
- ¼ cup sliced cucumbers
- ¼ avocado, sliced

Instructions:

1. Spread hummus on collard greens.
2. Add veggies and roll into wraps.

Fermented Veggie Quinoa Bowl

Ingredients:

- 1 cup cooked quinoa
- ½ cup fermented carrots (making instructions at the end of Recipes)
- ½ cup roasted sweet potatoes
- One tablespoon pumpkin seeds

Instructions:

1. Layer quinoa, veggies, and seeds in a bowl.
2. Drizzle with olive oil before serving.

DINNER RECIPES

Gut-Loving Lentil Stew

Ingredients:

- 1 cup cooked lentils
- ½ cup diced carrots
- ½ cup diced zucchini
- One tablespoon of miso paste
- 2 cups vegetable broth
- One teaspoon of turmeric powder

Instructions:

1. Sauté carrots and zucchini in a pot with a splash of olive oil.
2. Add lentils, broth, and turmeric. Simmer for 10 minutes.
3. Stir in miso paste just before serving to preserve probiotics.

Herb-crusted mackerel with Roasted Veggies

Ingredients:

- Two mackerel fillets (rich in omega-3s)
- One tablespoon of olive oil
- One teaspoon dried oregano
- One teaspoon of garlic powder
- 1 cup roasted Brussels sprouts and asparagus

Instructions:

1. Preheat oven to 375°F (190°C).
2. Brush mackerel fillets with olive oil and sprinkle with oregano and garlic powder.
3. Bake for 15–20 minutes. Serve with roasted veggies.

Ginger-Salmon Stir-Fry

Ingredients:

- 2 salmon fillets
- 1 cup broccoli florets
- 1 cup snap peas
- 1 teaspoon grated ginger
- 1 tablespoon coconut aminos

Instructions:

1. Sauté ginger in coconut oil.
2. Cook salmon and vegetables. Drizzle with coconut aminos.

Sweet Potato and Chickpea Curry

Ingredients:

- 1 cup diced sweet potatoes
- ½ cup cooked chickpeas
- 1 cup coconut milk
- 1 teaspoon curry powder

Instructions:

1. Sauté sweet potatoes and curry powder.
2. Add chickpeas and coconut milk. Simmer until tender.

Baked Cod with Herb Crust

Ingredients:

- 2 cod fillets
- 1 tablespoon olive oil
- 1 teaspoon dried thyme
- ½ cup roasted zucchini

Instructions:

1. Brush cod with olive oil and thyme.
2. Bake at 375°F for 15 minutes. Serve with zucchini.

Stuffed Bell Peppers

Ingredients:

- 2 bell peppers, halved
- 1 cup cooked quinoa
- ½ cup black beans
- 1 tablespoon tomato paste

Instructions:

1. Mix quinoa, beans, and tomato paste.
2. Stuff into peppers and bake at 375°F for 20 minutes.

Lentil and Spinach Soup

Ingredients:

- 1 cup cooked lentils
- 2 cups vegetable broth
- 1 cup fresh spinach
- 1 teaspoon cumin

Instructions:

1. Combine lentils and broth in a pot.
2. Add spinach and cumin. Simmer for 10 minutes.

SNACK RECIPES

Gut-Friendly Veggie Sticks with Hummus

Ingredients:

- One carrot, sliced into sticks
- One cucumber, sliced into sticks
- One red bell pepper, sliced
- ½ cup hummus (add a sprinkle of turmeric for anti-inflammatory benefits)

Instructions:

1. Arrange veggie sticks on a plate and serve with hummus.

Berry Kefir Smoothie

Ingredients:

- 1 cup plain kefir (or coconut kefir for dairy-free)
- ½ cup frozen mixed berries
- One tablespoon of chia seeds
- One teaspoon of honey or maple syrup

Instructions:

1. Blend all ingredients until smooth. Serve immediately.

Roasted Chickpeas

Ingredients:

- 1 cup canned chickpeas, rinsed and drained
- One teaspoon of olive oil
- ½ teaspoon smoked paprika

Instructions:

1. Toss chickpeas with olive oil and paprika.
2. Roast at 400°F for 20 minutes.

Nut Butter and Banana Bites

Ingredients:

- One banana, sliced
- Two tablespoons of almond or peanut butter

Instructions:

1. Spread nut butter between two banana slices.

Kimchi Deviled Eggs

Ingredients:

- Four boiled eggs, halved
- Two tablespoons kimchi, finely chopped
- One teaspoon Greek yogurt

Instructions:

1. Mash egg yolks with yogurt and kimchi.
2. Fill egg whites with the mixture.

Cucumber Dill Bites

Ingredients:

- One cucumber, sliced
- Two tablespoons of Greek yogurt
- One teaspoon of fresh dill

Instructions:

1. Top cucumber slices with yogurt and sprinkle with dill.

Dark Chocolate and Almond Bark

Ingredients:

- ½ cup dark chocolate (70% or higher)
- ¼ cup almonds, chopped

Instructions:

1. Melt chocolate and stir in almonds.
2. Spread on parchment paper and let cool before breaking into pieces.

OPTIONAL ADD-ONS

- Incorporate herbal teas like peppermint or chamomile to pair with these meals.
- Add fermented snacks like yogurt or tempeh to complement meals. (Tempeh details at the end of Recipes)

There are **healthy desserts** that promote **gut health wellness** as well, by incorporating ingredients that nourish the gut microbiome and support overall digestion. These desserts often include prebiotic fibers, probiotics, and anti-inflammatory ingredients. Here are some examples:

Greek Yogurt and Berry Parfait

Ingredients:

- 1 cup plain Greek yogurt (probiotic-rich)
- ½ cup mixed fresh berries (blueberries, raspberries, strawberries)
- One tablespoon of chia seeds (rich in fiber and omega-3s)
- 1 teaspoon honey or maple syrup

Instructions:

1. Layer yogurt, berries, and chia seeds in a glass.
2. Drizzle with honey or maple syrup.

Dark Chocolate Avocado Mousse

Ingredients:

- One ripe avocado
- Two tablespoons of unsweetened cocoa powder
- Two tablespoons of honey or maple syrup
- 1 teaspoon vanilla extract
- 1-2 tablespoons almond milk (as needed)

Instructions:

1. Blend all ingredients until smooth.
2. Chill in the refrigerator for 30 minutes before serving.

Chia Pudding

Ingredients:

- Three tablespoons chia seeds (prebiotic)
- 1 cup unsweetened almond or coconut milk
- ½ teaspoon vanilla extract
- One teaspoon of honey or maple syrup
- Optional toppings: fresh fruit, nuts, or granola

Instructions:

1. Mix chia seeds, milk, vanilla, and sweetener in a bowl.
2. Refrigerate for at least 4 hours (or overnight) until thickened.
3. Top with fruit or nuts before serving.

Fermented Coconut Yogurt with Granola

Ingredients:

- 1 cup coconut yogurt (probiotic-rich)
- ¼ cup homemade or low-sugar granola
- One tablespoon of shredded coconut
- A sprinkle of cinnamon

Instructions:

1. Spoon yogurt into a bowl.
2. Add granola, shredded coconut, and cinnamon on top.

Gut-Friendly Banana Bread

Ingredients:

- Two ripe bananas, mashed
- 1 cup almond flour
- 2 tablespoons ground flaxseed (fiber-rich)
- 2 eggs (or flax eggs for vegan)
- One teaspoon cinnamon
- 1 teaspoon baking powder
- Two tablespoons of honey or maple syrup
- ¼ cup chopped walnuts (optional)

Instructions:

1. Preheat oven to 350°F (175°C). Grease a loaf pan.
2. Mix all ingredients in a bowl until combined.
3. Pour into the pan and bake for 35-40 minutes.

Miso Caramel Apple Slices

Ingredients:

- One apple, sliced
- One tablespoon of miso paste
- Two tablespoons honey
- One tablespoon of almond butter

Instructions:

1. Mix miso, honey, and almond butter until smooth.
2. Drizzle over apple slices.

Probiotic Chocolate Bites

Ingredients:

- ½ cup dark chocolate (70% or higher)
- 2 tablespoons plain kefir (probiotic-rich)
- ¼ cup crushed almonds or hazelnuts

Instructions:

1. Melt the chocolate.
2. Stir in kefir and crushed nuts.
3. Pour into molds or a lined tray and refrigerate until firm.

Cinnamon Baked Pears

Ingredients:

- 2 ripe pears, halved and cored
- One teaspoon cinnamon
- One tablespoon honey
- One tablespoon of chopped walnuts (optional)

Instructions:

1. Preheat oven to 375°F (190°C).
2. Sprinkle pears with cinnamon and drizzle with honey.
3. Bake for 20 minutes and top with walnuts.

Gut-Healing Gummies

Ingredients:

- 1 cup kombucha (probiotic-rich)
- 1 tablespoon gelatin powder (supports gut lining)
- One teaspoon honey

Instructions:

1. Warm kombucha and stir in gelatin and honey.
2. Pour into molds and refrigerate until set.

Lemon Ginger Popsicles

Ingredients:

- One cup unsweetened coconut water
- Juice of 1 lemon
- One teaspoon of grated fresh ginger
- One teaspoon honey

Instructions:

1. Mix all ingredients and pour into popsicle molds.
2. Freeze for 4-6 hours.

MAKING FERMENTED CARROTS

Fermenting carrots is a simple and rewarding process that requires just a few basic ingredients and supplies. Here's a step-by-step guide to fermenting carrots:

Ingredients:

1. Fresh carrots (about 1–2 pounds)
2. Non-iodized salt (such as sea salt or kosher salt)
3. Filtered water (chlorine-free)
4. Optional: Flavorings like garlic, dill, ginger, or spices

Supplies:

- Mason jar or fermentation vessel
- A lid or fermentation weight (to keep the carrots submerged)
- A clean kitchen towel or airlock lid for fermentation

Instructions:

1. **Prepare the Carrots**

- Wash the carrots thoroughly to remove dirt. Peel them if desired, but leaving the skin can enhance fermentation because it contains natural bacteria.
- Cut the carrots into sticks, slices, or chunks, depending on your preference. Ensure they fit into your jar with some space at the top.

2. **Make the Brine**

- Dissolve one tablespoon of salt in 2 cups of filtered water. The salt-to-water ratio should be approximately 2–3% by weight, which is ideal for fermentation.

3. **Pack the Jar**

- Place the carrots into the jar tightly but without crushing them.
- If using flavorings, layer them with the carrots for an extra burst of flavor.

4. **Add the Brine**

- Pour the brine over the carrots until they are completely submerged. Leave about 1 inch of headspace at the top of the jar to allow for expansion during fermentation.

5. **Weigh Down the Carrots**

- Use a fermentation weight or a small, clean object (like a smaller jar or a sterilized rock) to keep the carrots submerged under the brine. This prevents mold and ensures proper fermentation.

6. **Cover the Jar**

- Cover the jar with a lid, fermentation airlock, or a clean kitchen towel secured with a rubber band. If using a regular lid, you may need to "burp" the jar daily to release gas buildup.

7. **Ferment**

- Place the jar in a cool, dark place (around 65–75°F/18–24°C) to ferment.
- Taste the carrots after 3–5 days and continue fermenting until they reach your desired flavor and tanginess. This

may take 7–14 days or longer, depending on temperature and personal preference.

8. **Store the Fermented Carrots**

- Once the carrots are fermented to your liking, transfer the jar to the refrigerator to slow the fermentation process. They can be stored for several months.

Tips:

- Use clean utensils each time you taste the carrots to avoid introducing unwanted bacteria.
- Watch for bubbling or a slight cloudiness in the brine—this is normal and indicates active fermentation.
- If mold develops on the surface, carefully remove it. The carrots below the brine are usually safe.

Enjoy your tangy, flavorful fermented carrots as a snack, in salads, or as a topping for various dishes!

MAKING SAUERKRAUT

Ingredients:

- 1 medium head of green or red cabbage (about 2 pounds)
- 1–2 tablespoons non-iodized salt (sea salt or kosher salt)
- Optional: Caraway seeds, juniper berries, or other spices for flavor

Supplies:

- Large bowl
- Mason jar or fermentation crock
- Fermentation weight or a smaller jar for pressing the cabbage
- Lid or cloth cover with a rubber band

Instructions:

1. **Prepare the Cabbage**
   - Remove outer leaves, and set one large leaf aside.
   - Slice the cabbage into thin strips or shred it with a food processor.
2. **Salt the Cabbage**
   - Place the cabbage in a large bowl and sprinkle with salt.
   - Massage the cabbage for about 5–10 minutes until it softens and releases liquid (brine).
3. **Pack the Jar**
   - Pack the salted cabbage tightly into a clean mason jar or crock. Use a spoon or your fist to press it down, ensuring the brine covers the cabbage.
4. **Add a Weight**
   - Place the reserved cabbage leaf on top and use a fermentation weight (or a smaller jar filled with water) to keep the cabbage submerged in the brine.
5. **Cover the Jar**
   - Cover the jar with a lid, airlock, or clean cloth secured with a rubber band.
6. **Ferment**
   - Let the jar sit at room temperature (65–75°F/18–24°C) for 1–4 weeks. Taste the sauerkraut after 5–7 days and ferment until you reach your preferred tanginess.

7. **Store**
    - Once fermented, transfer the sauerkraut to the refrigerator. It will keep for several months.

MAKING KIMCHI

Ingredients:

- 1 medium napa cabbage (about 2 pounds)
- 1/4 cup non-iodized salt
- 1–2 tablespoons fish sauce (optional)
- 1–2 tablespoons Korean red chili flakes (gochugaru)
- 1 tablespoon minced garlic
- 1 teaspoon minced ginger
- 2 teaspoons sugar
- 4–5 green onions, chopped
- Optional: 1/2 cup julienned carrots or daikon radish

Supplies:

- Large bowl
- Mason jar or fermentation crock
- Fermentation weight or a smaller jar
- Lid or cloth cover with a rubber band

Instructions:

1. **Prepare the Cabbage**
    - Cut the napa cabbage into quarters, then chop it into bite-sized pieces.
    - In a large bowl, sprinkle salt over the cabbage and massage gently. Add water to cover the cabbage and let it sit for 1–2 hours.

2. **Rinse the Cabbage**
   - Drain and rinse the cabbage thoroughly to remove excess salt. Set aside.
3. **Make the Kimchi Paste**
   - In a small bowl, mix the fish sauce, chili flakes, garlic, ginger, sugar, and optional vegetables (carrots or daikon).
4. **Combine**
   - Add the kimchi paste to the cabbage and green onions. Use gloves to massage the paste into the cabbage until evenly coated.
5. **Pack the Jar**
   - Pack the kimchi tightly into a mason jar or crock. Press it down to ensure the brine rises to cover the cabbage.
6. **Add a Weight**
   - Place a fermentation weight or small jar on top to keep the kimchi submerged in the brine.
7. **Cover the Jar**
   - Cover the jar with a lid, airlock, or cloth secured with a rubber band.
8. **Ferment**
   - Let the jar sit at room temperature for 2–5 days. Check daily to release gas, and press the cabbage down if needed.
9. **Store**
   - Once fermented to your liking, transfer the kimchi to the refrigerator. It will keep for several months.

Tips for Both Sauerkraut and Kimchi:

- Ensure all vegetables stay submerged in the brine to prevent mold.
- Use clean utensils each time you taste or adjust.

- Fermentation time can vary based on temperature and taste preferences.

Enjoy your homemade fermented creations as side dishes, toppings, or snacks!

TEMPEH AND ITS KEY FEATURES

Tempeh is a traditional Indonesian food made by **fermenting cooked soybeans**. It is formed into a compact cake or block and is prized for its high protein content, nutty flavor, and versatility. It is an excellent plant-based protein source, making it popular in vegetarian and vegan diets.

1. **Main Ingredient**:
   - Tempeh is typically made from soybeans but can also include other legumes, grains (like rice or barley), or seeds.
2. **Fermentation Process**:
   - Cooked soybeans are inoculated with a specific fungus, *Rhizopus oligosporus*.
   - The fungus ferments the soybeans, binding them to a firm, cake-like texture.
3. **Nutritional Benefits**:
   - **Protein**: A great source of complete protein, containing all essential amino acids.
   - **Fiber**: High in dietary fiber, supporting gut health.
   - **Probiotics**: The fermentation process may introduce beneficial probiotics, aiding digestion.
   - **Rich in Nutrients**: Contains iron, calcium, magnesium, and B vitamins, including B12 in fortified versions.

4. **Flavor and Texture**:
   - Tempeh has a nutty, earthy taste with a firm and chewy texture. The flavor can be mild, which makes it absorb marinades and seasonings well.
5. **Versatility**:
   - Tempeh can be grilled, sautéed, baked, crumbled, or steamed. It's often used as a meat substitute in stir-fries, salads, sandwiches, or tacos.

HEALTH BENEFITS OF TEMPEH

- **Heart Health**: It contains healthy fats and no cholesterol, making it heart-friendly.
- **Gut Health**: Fermented food may support a healthy microbiome.
- **Bone Health**: High calcium content helps maintain strong bones.
- **Weight Management**: Low in carbs and high in protein, aiding satiety.
- **Antioxidants**: Contains natural antioxidants from the fermentation process.

TEMPEH VS. TOFU

- **Texture**: Tempeh is firmer and chewier, while tofu is softer and smoother.
- **Flavor**: Tempeh has a nutty, robust flavor, while tofu is relatively bland and neutral.
- **Processing**: Tempeh is fermented, while tofu is made by coagulating soy milk.

Tempeh is a nutritious, versatile food that works well in a variety of dishes, providing both flavor and health benefits!

MAKING TEMPEH

Making tempeh at home involves fermenting soybeans with a specific fungus (*Rhizopus oligosporus*). The process requires clean conditions, patience, and attention to temperature. Here's a step-by-step guide:

Ingredients:

- **2 cups dried soybeans**
- **1 tablespoon white vinegar** (to lower the pH for fermentation)
- **1 teaspoon tempeh starter culture** (*Rhizopus oligosporus* spores, available online or in specialty stores)

Equipment:

- Large bowl for soaking
- Large pot for cooking
- Colander for draining
- A clean towel or cheesecloth
- Baking dish or plastic bag with small holes (for fermentation)
- Incubator or warm spot to maintain 86–90°F (30–32°C)

Instructions:

Prepare the Soybeans:

- Rinse the soybeans to remove any debris.
- **Soak** the beans in water overnight (12–18 hours).

- After soaking, **dehull** the soybeans by rubbing them between your hands. This helps remove their outer skins, which can inhibit fermentation. (Removing all the hulls isn't necessary, but it's ideal for better results.)
- Rinse the beans thoroughly to remove the loosened hulls.

Cook the Soybeans:

- Boil the dehulled soybeans in fresh water for about 30 minutes until they are cooked but not mushy.
- Drain the beans well and transfer them to a clean towel to dry. Excess moisture can hinder fermentation.

Acidify the Beans:

- Add **one tablespoon of vinegar** to the beans and mix well. This lowers the pH, which prevents unwanted bacteria growth.

Inoculate the Beans:

- Let the beans cool to about 95–105°F (35–40°C) before adding the tempeh starter.
- Sprinkle **one teaspoon of tempeh starter** evenly over the beans.
- Mix thoroughly to ensure even distribution of the spores.

Prepare for Fermentation:

- Transfer the inoculated soybeans into a clean plastic bag or shallow container. If using a plastic bag, **poke small holes** every 2 inches to allow airflow during fermentation.

- Flatten the beans into an even layer about 1 inch thick. This ensures proper fermentation.

Ferment the Tempeh:

- Place the filled container or bag in an incubator or warm spot where you can maintain a steady temperature of 86–90°F (30–32°C).
- Allow the beans to ferment for **24–48 hours**. Check periodically to ensure the temperature remains stable.
- After 12–24 hours, white mycelium begins to grow, binding the beans together into a firm cake.

Check and Store:

- After 48 hours, the tempeh should have a solid texture and a white, fuzzy appearance. It may have a light nutty or mushroom-like smell, which is normal.
- Stop the fermentation by storing the tempeh in the refrigerator or freezer.

Tips for Success:

- **Cleanliness is critical**: Ensure all tools and surfaces are sanitized to avoid contamination.
- **Monitor temperature closely**: Tempeh thrives in a warm, humid environment. Too high or low a temperature can disrupt fermentation.
- **Be patient**: The process takes time, but the result is worth the wait!

HOW TO USE HOMEMADE TEMPEH:

- **Cook It First**: Steam, fry, or bake tempeh before consuming. This enhances the flavor and makes it more digestible.
- **Recipes**: Use it in stir-fries, sandwiches, tacos, salads, or as a meat substitute.

This is more than just a sample week of nutritious meals; it's a stepping stone toward long-term transformation. Your journey to gut-brain wellness is an evolving process. Use this plan as a foundation, and feel free to adapt it to your preferences and lifestyle. Experiment with flavors, discover new ingredients, and make it uniquely yours. The more you enjoy the process, the more sustainable it becomes.

SHARE YOUR REVIEW AND HELP FELLOW READERS!

We hope you've enjoyed "THE GUT-BRAIN CONNECTION - A HOLISTIC APPROACH" by N.R. Sterling. Your journey towards living your best life is just beginning, and your feedback can make a big difference.

How You Can Help:

- **Share Your Experience:** What did you love about the book? Did a specific chapter or tip stand out and help you?
- **Keep It Simple:** A few sentences about what you liked and how the book helped you is perfect
- **Be Honest:** Your genuine opinion helps us improve and guide other readers.
- **Why It Matters:** Your review is crucial. It helps others decide if this book is right for them and enables us to create better content for future readers like you.

Thank you for being part of our community and helping us make this book the best it can be!

Scan the QR code to leave a review.

CONCLUSION

So, here we are, at the end of our journey through the fascinating world of the gut-brain connection. You've likely gathered by now that understanding and nurturing this axis is a vital component of overall well-being. The gut and brain are in constant conversation, influencing everything from your mood to how you digest your morning coffee. This bidirectional communication impacts your physical, mental, and emotional health in profound ways.

Throughout this book, we have emphasized the significance of adopting a holistic approach to wellness. We've explored how diet, lifestyle, and stress management play pivotal roles in maintaining a healthy gut. You've seen how stress can turn your gut into a battleground and how a diverse microbiome can be your best defense. Because this interconnectedness of stress and gut health affects both ways, we are including a final summary of stress management techniques for easy reference. Each technique works differently for everyone, so experimenting with what resonates most can lead to a personalized stress-relief toolkit.

Physical Techniques

1. **Brisk Walks or Jogging**: Walking releases endorphins, improves circulation, and provides a mental break, helping to reduce stress and clear your mind. Nature walks or walking in green spaces can have an even greater calming effect.
2. **Strength Training**: Weightlifting or resistance exercises can help channel stress and improve overall mood by boosting endorphins and reducing tension.
3. **Dancing**: Moving to music can be both a physical release and a fun distraction, lifting your spirits and lowering stress.
4. **Stretching**: Even if it's not a full yoga session, simple stretches can help release muscle tension and promote relaxation.
5. **Swimming**: The rhythmic movement of swimming and being in water can be incredibly soothing for the body and mind.

Creative Outlets

1. **Art Therapy**: Drawing, painting, or coloring (e.g., in an adult coloring book) can help you express emotions and feel more relaxed.
2. **Playing Music**: Whether it's learning an instrument or simply enjoying your favorite songs, music can significantly lower stress levels.
3. **Writing or Journaling**: Putting your thoughts on paper helps process emotions and gain clarity, reducing mental overload.
4. **Crafting**: Activities like knitting, pottery, or scrapbooking provide a focus and calming rhythm that can lower stress.

Social Techniques

1. **Talking to a Friend**: A trusted friend or loved one can help you vent, feel heard, and gain perspective.
2. **Joining a Group Activity**: Whether it's a book club, sports team, or hobby group, shared experiences can reduce feelings of isolation.
3. **Laughter Therapy**: Watching a funny movie, stand-up comedy, or even laughing with friends can release stress-busting endorphins.

Sensory Techniques

1. **Deep Breathing Exercises**: Practicing diaphragmatic breathing can calm the nervous system and bring you back to the present moment.
2. **Aromatherapy**: Essential oils like lavender, chamomile, or eucalyptus can create a relaxing atmosphere.
3. **Warm Baths or Showers**: The soothing effects of warm water can reduce muscle tension and calm your mind.

Mindful Activities

1. **Gardening**: Working with plants can be meditative, connect you to nature, and provide a sense of accomplishment.
2. **Cooking or Baking**: Creating meals can be both a sensory and grounding activity that reduces stress while nourishing your body.
3. **Puzzles and Brain Games**: Activities like jigsaw puzzles, Sudoku, or crosswords provide mental engagement and relaxation.

Lifestyle Adjustments

1. **Reading**: Immersing yourself in a good book can provide an escape and reduce stress.
2. **Prioritizing Sleep**: Getting enough quality rest helps your body recover and better handle stress.
3. **Digital Detox**: Taking breaks from screens and social media helps lower overstimulation and mental fatigue.
4. **Time Management**: Organizing your day with lists or schedules can help reduce the feeling of being overwhelmed.
5. **Volunteering**: Helping others fosters gratitude and shifts your focus away from stress.

Outdoor Activities

1. **Gardening or Plant Care**: Connecting with nature, even in your backyard, can soothe the mind.
2. **Cycling**: It has low impact and is rhythmic; it's a great way to get outside and release tension.
3. **Playing with Pets**: Spending time with animals can naturally lower stress hormones like cortisol.

Stress Management for Immediate Relief

1. **Progressive Muscle Relaxation**: Tense and release each muscle group to relieve physical stress.
2. **Chewing Gum**: A surprising stress reliever, chewing gum can reduce cortisol levels and improve focus.
3. **Sipping Herbal Tea**: Calming teas like chamomile or peppermint can help you unwind.

Remember all the practical strategies we discussed throughout the book? They're your toolkit for nurturing the gut-brain axis.

Now, here's where you come in. This journey is about taking action. Start incorporating the practices we've discussed into your life. Whether it's experimenting with a new dietary plan, trying out a stress-reduction technique, or exploring natural remedies, every small step counts. Embracing these holistic health practices fosters personal growth and improves your well-being.

Stay curious and keep learning because the science of gut-brain health is evolving, and new insights are constantly emerging. Be open-minded and adaptable; your health journey is a process, and continuous learning is key to staying on track.

As you move forward, carry with you the understanding that your gut and brain are powerful allies. Treat them well, and they'll support you in ways you never imagined. Here's to a future filled with health, happiness, and harmony. Keep nurturing that gut-brain connection, and it will lead you to a life of well-being and fulfillment.

REFERENCES

National Center for Biotechnology Information. (n.d.). *The gut-brain axis: Interactions between enteric microbiota.* Retrieved from https://pmc.ncbi.nlm.nih.gov/articles/PMC4367209/

Scientific American. (n.d.). *Think twice: How the gut's "second brain" influences mood and well-being.* Retrieved from https://www.scientificamerican.com/article/gut-second-brain/

CAS. (n.d.). *How your gut microbiome is linked to depression and anxiety.* Retrieved from https://www.cas.org/resources/cas-insights/how-your-gut-microbiome-linked-depression-and-anxiety

Healthline. (n.d.). *The gut-brain connection: How it works and the role of nutrition.* Retrieved from https://www.healthline.com/nutrition/gut-brain-connection

Health. (n.d.). *Holistic health: Definition, benefits, tips.* Retrieved from https://www.health.com/holistic-health-8652522

WFLA. (n.d.). *The science behind holistic healing: Uniting body, mind, and soul.* Retrieved from https://www.wfla.com/bloom-tampa-bay/the-science-behind-holistic-healing-uniting-body-mind-and-soul/

Healthline. (n.d.). *Can yoga help aid digestion? 9 poses to try.* Retrieved from https://www.healthline.com/nutrition/yoga-posture-for-digestion

National Center for Biotechnology Information. (n.d.). *Gut microbiota and neuroplasticity.* Retrieved from https://pmc.ncbi.nlm.nih.gov/articles/PMC8392499/

Healthline. (n.d.). *Probiotics and prebiotics: What's the difference?.* Retrieved from https://www.healthline.com/nutrition/probiotics-and-prebiotics

National Center for Biotechnology Information. (n.d.). *Fermented foods, health, and the gut microbiome.* Retrieved from https://pmc.ncbi.nlm.nih.gov/articles/PMC9003261/

Ruscio, M. (n.d.). *How to target neuroinflammation and beat brain fog.* Retrieved from https://drruscio.com/neuroinflammation/

Harvard Health Publishing. (2015). *Nutritional psychiatry: Your brain on food.* Retrieved from https://www.health.harvard.edu/blog/nutritional-psychiatry-your-brain-on-food-201511168626

Herbazest. (n.d.). *Improving gut-brain axis with herbs.* Retrieved from https://www.herbazest.com/wellness/improving-gut-brain-axis-with-herbs

National Center for Biotechnology Information. (n.d.). *Anti-inflammatory effects of curcumin in the gut microbiome*. Retrieved from https://pmc.ncbi.nlm.nih.gov/articles/PMC8572027/

ScienceDirect. (n.d.). *The effect of adaptogenic plants on stress: A systematic review*. Retrieved from https://www.sciencedirect.com/science/article/pii/S1756464623002955

National Center for Biotechnology Information. (n.d.). *Effects of probiotics, prebiotics, and synbiotics on human health*. Retrieved from https://pmc.ncbi.nlm.nih.gov/articles/PMC5622781/

National Center for Biotechnology Information. (n.d.). *Posttraumatic stress disorder: Does the gut microbiome hold the key?*. Retrieved from https://pmc.ncbi.nlm.nih.gov/articles/PMC4794957/

National Center for Biotechnology Information. (n.d.). *Posttraumatic stress disorder: Does the gut microbiome hold the key?*. Retrieved from https://pmc.ncbi.nlm.nih.gov/articles/PMC4794957/

National Center for Biotechnology Information. (n.d.). *Microbial reprogramming in obsessive–compulsive disorders*. Retrieved from https://pmc.ncbi.nlm.nih.gov/articles/PMC10419219/

Gut Pathogens. (n.d.). *Strain-specific effects of probiotics on depression and anxiety*. Retrieved from https://gutpathogens.biomedcentral.com/articles/10.1186/s13099-024-00634-8

Microbiome Journal. (n.d.). *Gut dysbiosis induces the development of depression-like behavior*. Retrieved from https://microbiomejournal.biomedcentral.com/articles/10.1186/s40168-024-01756-6

National Center for Biotechnology Information. (n.d.). *Current evidence on the role of the gut microbiome in health and disease*. Retrieved from https://pmc.ncbi.nlm.nih.gov/articles/PMC7830868/

BMC Medicine. (n.d.). *Mediterranean diet adherence is associated with lower depression risk*. Retrieved from https://bmcmedicine.biomedcentral.com/articles/10.1186/s12916-023-02772-3

Nature. (n.d.). *Microbiota–gut–brain axis mechanisms in the complex regulation of behavior*. Retrieved from https://www.nature.com/articles/s41380-023-01964-w

National Center for Biotechnology Information. (n.d.). *The relationship between gut microbiota and insomnia*. Retrieved from https://pmc.ncbi.nlm.nih.gov/articles/PMC10714008/

National Center for Biotechnology Information. (n.d.). *The dynamic interplay between the gut microbiota and immune function*. Retrieved from https://pmc.ncbi.nlm.nih.gov/articles/PMC6854958/

Healthline. (n.d.). *AIP (Autoimmune Protocol) diet: A beginner's guide*. Retrieved from https://www.healthline.com/nutrition/aip-diet-autoimmune-protocol-diet

Restorative Medicine Journal. (n.d.). *Natural support for autoimmune and inflammatory disease*. Retrieved from https://restorativemedicine.org/journal/natural-support-for-autoimmune-and-inflammatory-disease/

National Center for Biotechnology Information. (n.d.). *A combination of healthy lifestyle behaviors reduces the risk of chronic disease*. Retrieved from https://pmc.ncbi.nlm.nih.gov/articles/PMC8792100/

National Center for Biotechnology Information. (n.d.). *Irritable bowel syndrome and the gut microbiome*. Retrieved from https://pmc.ncbi.nlm.nih.gov/articles/PMC10095554/

Healthline. (n.d.). *Does gluten cause leaky gut syndrome?*. Retrieved from https://www.healthline.com/nutrition/gluten-leaky-gut

National Center for Biotechnology Information. (n.d.). *Impact of the gut microbiota on the development of obesity*. Retrieved from https://pmc.ncbi.nlm.nih.gov/articles/PMC4010744/

Harvard Medical School. (n.d.). *Gut-brain connection in autism*. Retrieved from https://hms.harvard.edu/news/gut-brain-connection-autism

WebMD. (n.d.). *Dysbiosis: Gut imbalance, IBD, and more*. Retrieved from https://www.webmd.com/digestive-disorders/what-is-dysbiosis

Harvard Health Publishing. (n.d.). *The gut-brain connection*. Retrieved from https://www.health.harvard.edu/diseases-and-conditions/the-gut-brain-connection

National Center for Biotechnology Information. (n.d.). *The role of gut microbiome in inflammatory skin disorders*. Retrieved from https://pmc.ncbi.nlm.nih.gov/articles/PMC8969879/

National Center for Biotechnology Information. (n.d.). *Gut microbiota's effect on mental health: The gut-brain axis*. Retrieved from https://pmc.ncbi.nlm.nih.gov/articles/PMC5641835/

The Times of India. (n.d.). *5 superb ways to detox and cleanse the gut*. Retrieved from https://timesofindia.indiatimes.com/life-style/health-fitness/health-news/5-superb-ways-to-detox-and-cleanse-the-gut/articleshow/113695221.cms

Glacier Fresh. (n.d.). *Detoxification and hydration: How water supports the body's natural cleansing processes*. Retrieved from https://glacierfreshfilter.com/blogs/news/detoxification-and-hydration-how-water-supports-the-bodys-natural-cleansing-processes

GoodTherapy. (n.d.). *How to go on a true mental detox in 7 steps*. Retrieved from https://www.goodtherapy.org/blog/True-Mental-Detox

News-Medical. (n.d.). *The effect of intermittent fasting on the gut microbiome*. Retrieved from https://www.news-medical.net/health/The-Effect-of-Intermittent-Fasting-on-the-Gut-Microbiome.aspx

REFERENCES

Healthline. (n.d.). *AIP (Autoimmune Protocol) diet: A beginner's guide*. Retrieved from https://www.healthline.com/nutrition/aip-diet-autoimmune-protocol-diet

Restorative Medicine Journal. (n.d.). *Natural support for autoimmune and inflammatory disease*. Retrieved from https://restorativemedicine.org/journal/natural-support-for-autoimmune-and-inflammatory-disease/

National Center for Biotechnology Information. (n.d.). *A combination of healthy lifestyle behaviors reduces the risk of chronic disease*. Retrieved from https://pmc.ncbi.nlm.nih.gov/articles/PMC8792100/

National Center for Biotechnology Information. (n.d.). *Irritable bowel syndrome and the gut microbiome*. Retrieved from https://pmc.ncbi.nlm.nih.gov/articles/PMC10095554/

Healthline. (n.d.). *Does gluten cause leaky gut syndrome?*. Retrieved from https://www.healthline.com/nutrition/gluten-leaky-gut

National Center for Biotechnology Information. (n.d.). *Impact of the gut microbiota on the development of obesity*. Retrieved from https://pmc.ncbi.nlm.nih.gov/articles/PMC4010744/

Harvard Medical School. (n.d.). *Gut-brain connection in autism*. Retrieved from https://hms.harvard.edu/news/gut-brain-connection-autism

WebMD. (n.d.). *Dysbiosis: Gut imbalance, IBD, and more*. Retrieved from https://www.webmd.com/digestive-disorders/what-is-dysbiosis

Harvard Health Publishing. (n.d.). *The gut-brain connection*. Retrieved from https://www.health.harvard.edu/diseases-and-conditions/the-gut-brain-connection

National Center for Biotechnology Information. (n.d.). *The role of gut microbiome in inflammatory skin disorders*. Retrieved from https://pmc.ncbi.nlm.nih.gov/articles/PMC8969879/

National Center for Biotechnology Information. (n.d.). *Gut microbiota's effect on mental health: The gut-brain axis*. Retrieved from https://pmc.ncbi.nlm.nih.gov/articles/PMC5641835/

The Times of India. (n.d.). *5 superb ways to detox and cleanse the gut*. Retrieved from https://timesofindia.indiatimes.com/life-style/health-fitness/health-news/5-superb-ways-to-detox-and-cleanse-the-gut/articleshow/113695221.cms

Glacier Fresh. (n.d.). *Detoxification and hydration: How water supports the body's natural cleansing processes*. Retrieved from https://glacierfreshfilter.com/blogs/news/detoxification-and-hydration-how-water-supports-the-bodys-natural-cleansing-processes

GoodTherapy. (n.d.). *How to go on a true mental detox in 7 steps*. Retrieved from https://www.goodtherapy.org/blog/True-Mental-Detox

News-Medical. (n.d.). *The effect of intermittent fasting on the gut microbiome*. Retrieved from https://www.news-medical.net/health/The-Effect-of-Intermittent-Fasting-on-the-Gut-Microbiome.aspx

National Center for Biotechnology Information. (n.d.). *Exercise modifies the gut microbiota with positive health effects.* Retrieved from https://pmc.ncbi.nlm.nih.gov/articles/PMC5357536/

Move Therapy and Wellness. (n.d.). *Mind your gut: Mindfulness for gastrointestinal diseases.* Retrieved from https://movetherapyandwellness.com/mind-your-gut-mindfulness-for-gastrointestinal-diseases/

Eco Modern Essentials. (n.d.). *Essential oils for emotional health.* Retrieved from https://ecomodernessentials.com.au/blogs/eco-modern-essentials-blog/essential-oils-for-emotional-balance

National Center for Biotechnology Information. (n.d.). *Exercise for mental health.* Retrieved from https://pmc.ncbi.nlm.nih.gov/articles/PMC1470658/

National Center for Biotechnology Information. (n.d.). *Signaling cognition: The gut microbiota and hypothalamic interactions.* Retrieved from https://pmc.ncbi.nlm.nih.gov/articles/PMC10316519/

The Beauty Chef. (n.d.). *How cortisol affects gut health and the microbiome.* Retrieved from https://thebeautychef.com/blogs/articles/how-cortisol-affects-gut-health-and-the-microbiome

American Psychological Association. (n.d.). *Mindfulness meditation: A research-proven way to reduce stress.* Retrieved from https://www.apa.org/topics/mindfulness/meditation

National Center for Biotechnology Information. (n.d.). *Associations between nature exposure and health.* Retrieved from https://pmc.ncbi.nlm.nih.gov/articles/PMC8125471/

Healthline. (n.d.). *How does your gut microbiome impact your overall health?.* Retrieved from https://www.healthline.com/nutrition/gut-microbiome-and-health

National Center for Biotechnology Information. (n.d.). *Impact of environmental pollutants on the gut microbiome.* Retrieved from https://pmc.ncbi.nlm.nih.gov/articles/PMC9317668/

ScienceDirect. (n.d.). *Antibiotics and the gut microbiome: Understanding the impact.* Retrieved from https://www.sciencedirect.com/science/article/pii/S2590097824000090

Gut Microbiota for Health. (n.d.). *Practical recommendations to increase gut microbial diversity.* Retrieved from https://www.gutmicrobiotaforhealth.com/practical-recommendations-to-increase-gut-microbial-diversity/

Medical News Today. (n.d.). *What to know about microbiome testing.* Retrieved from https://www.medicalnewstoday.com/articles/microbiome-testing

ScienceDirect. (n.d.). *Tracking a dysregulated gut-brain axis with biomarkers.* Retrieved from https://www.sciencedirect.com/science/article/pii/S2666144619300097

National Center for Biotechnology Information. (n.d.). *Making health habitual: The psychology of 'habit-formation'*. Retrieved from https://pmc.ncbi.nlm.nih.gov/articles/PMC3505409/

Serenity Wellness and Counseling. (n.d.). *How integrative health practitioners tailor treatments to help the gut and improve mental health disorders*. Retrieved from https://serenitywellnessandcounseling.com/personalized-wellness-plans-how-integrative-health-practitioners-tailor-treatments-to-help-the-gut-and-improve-mental-health-disorders/

MyBioPedia. (n.d.). *Herbs to improve memory: 4 herbs everyone needs*. Retrieved from https://www.mybiopedia.com/4-herbs-to-improve-memory-brain-health-and-cognitive-function

The Bed Sheets Club. (n.d.). *9 best herbs for sleep: Boosting your sleep quality naturally*. Retrieved from https://thebedsheetclub.com/blogs/the-bed-sheet-club/10-best-herbs-for-sleep-boosting-your-sleep-quality-naturally

The Rike. (n.d.). *Mastering the art of brewing herbal tea*. Retrieved from https://therike.com/blogs/self-cure-herbal-medicine-home-natural-remedy/discover-the-secrets-to-brewing-perfect-cup-of-herbal-tea

Dr. Berg. (n.d.). *Good bacteria keep Candida, fungus, and yeast in check*. Retrieved from https://www.drberg.com/blog/good-bacteria-keep-candida-fungus-and-yeast-in-check

BioTurmric. (n.d.). *Natural supplements for promoting gut health and digestion*. Retrieved from https://bioturmric.com/de/blogs/news/natural-supplements-for-promoting-gut-health-and-digestion

Xaviax. (n.d.). *Complete gut health: Unlocking the key to wellness*. Retrieved from https://xaviax.com/blogs/probiotic-news/complete-gut-health

Shield Vitamins. (n.d.). *Prebiotics vs probiotics: Decoding the differences and how they impact your health*. Retrieved from https://shieldvitamins.com/blogs/articles/prebiotics-vs-probiotics-decoding-the-differences

Just Add Buoy. (n.d.). *Exploring the health benefits of magnesium: A comprehensive guide*. Retrieved from https://justaddbuoy.com/blogs/hydration-station/health-benefits-magnesium

Dr. Maggie Yu. (n.d.). *Best probiotics for autoimmune disease*. Retrieved from https://drmaggieyu.com/blog/best-probiotics-for-autoimmune-disease/

Productcaster. (n.d.). *Probiotic capsules: Containing prebiotics and digestive enzymes*. Retrieved from https://css.productcaster.com/fi/product/flash-sale-naisten-lyhyt-mp-tempo-ultra-takki-deep-lagoon-m-8cb12b4d-f0fc-47ad-b4cb-64ba122bce62/

Such Science. (n.d.). *Best sea moss capsules: Top picks for optimal health benefits*. Retrieved from https://suchscience.net/best-sea-moss-capsules/

Flourish Pharmacy & Nutrition. (n.d.). *6 benefits of natural supplements*. Retrieved from https://flourishrx.com/6-benefits-of-natural-supplements/

REFERENCES • 187

All Good Health. (n.d.). *Should you take phosphatidylserine and ashwagandha together?*. Retrieved from https://allgoodhealth.net/nootropics/should-you-take-phosphatidylserine-and-ashwagandha-together/

Ekaa Kombucha. (n.d.). *Gut health reimagined: Why your gut matters and how Ekaa Kombucha can help*. Retrieved from https://ekaakombucha.com/gut-health-reimagined-why-your-gut-matters-and-how-ekaa-kombucha-can-help/

Revival Point. (n.d.). *Unveiling the power of resistant starches: Boosting gut health and nutrient absorption*. Retrieved from https://revivalpoint.com/a/blog/unveiling-the-power-of-resistant-starches-boosting-gut-health-and-nutrient-absorption

Social Moms. (2024). *Best supplement to prevent gas and bloating (2024 update)*. Retrieved from https://www.socialmoms.com/featured/best-supplement-to-prevent-gas-and-bloating/

GutHealth.org. (n.d.). *Top types of gut health supplements*. Retrieved from https://guthealth.org/supplements-gut-health/

Nutri Guide. (2018). *Fermented vegetables for a healthy gut*. Retrieved from https://nutri.guide/2018/11/08/fermented-vegetables-for-a-healthy-gut/

Ero Texas. (n.d.). *Cooked or raw? The best ways to eat 9 healthy veggies*. Retrieved from https://www.eroftexas.com/best-ways-to-eat-9-healthy-veggies-cooked-raw/

Cerritos Community News. (2024). *Probiotics: A guide to support gut health*. Retrieved from https://www.loscerritosnews.net/2024/07/30/probiotics-a-guide-to-support-gut-health/

Gochujar Global. (n.d.). *[CKD] Lacto-Fit Probiotics GOLD*. Retrieved from https://global.gochujar.com/collections/most-recently-purchased/products/ckd-lacto-fit-probiotics-gold

Probiotics Everything. (n.d.). *Fermentation fascination: Exploring fermented foods and their probiotic punch*. Retrieved from https://probioticseverything.com/fermentation-fascination-exploring-fermented-foods-and-their-probiotic-punch/

Trtl Health. (n.d.). *Brain fog: Causes, tests, solutions*. Retrieved from https://trtl.health/blogs/news/trtl-health-brain-fog-causes-tests

Lifestyle Clinic. (n.d.). *Can food affect my heart health?*. Retrieved from https://www.lifestyle-clinic.com/post/can-food-affect-my-heart-health

The Gut Doc. (n.d.). *Herbal remedies for gut problems*. Retrieved from https://thegutdoc.net/herbal-remedies-for-gut-problems/

Brave in Bloom. (n.d.). *Discover the best anti-aging vegetables to add to your diet*. Retrieved from https://braveinbloom.com/blogs/anti-aging-journal/discover-the-best-anti-aging-vegetables-to-add-to-your-diet

Health Blog Centre Info. (n.d.). *Do probiotics really benefit healthy people?*. Retrieved from http://yourhealthblog.net/do-probiotics-really-benefit-healthy-people/

Nutrition4Kids. (n.d.). *Prebiotics, probiotics, and synbiotics: Promoting our health*. Retrieved from https://nutrition4kids.com/articles/prebiotics-probiotics-and-synbiotics-promoting-our-health/

Psych Central. (n.d.). *What to know about OCD: Symptoms, causes, treatment.* Retrieved from https://psychcentral.com/ocd/ocd-overview

Medical News Daily. (2023). *Navigating the future: Anxiety research in fall 2023.* Retrieved from https://www.medicalnewsdaily.com/navigating-the-future-anxiety-research-in-fall-2023/

HealthyZo. (n.d.). *How to improve gut health and reduce stress naturally: A comprehensive guide.* Retrieved from https://healthyzo.com/blog/how-to-improve-gut-health-and-reduce-stress-naturally-a-comprehensive-approach/

MyHealthBooster. (n.d.). *Nourishing the mind: Foods that boost mental wellness.* Retrieved from https://www.myhealthbooster.com/title-nourishing-the-mind-foods-that-boost-mental-wellness/

Lotus on Main. (n.d.). *What is the science behind the mind-body connection?.* Retrieved from https://lotusonmain.com/what-is-the-science-behind-the-mind-body-connection/

Psychreg. (n.d.). *Altered gut microbes may affect risk of ADHD.* Retrieved from https://www.psychreg.org/altered-gut-microbes-may-affect-risk-adhd/

Internet Vibes. (2023). *5 best supplements to add to your daily wellness routine.* Retrieved from https://www.internetvibes.net/2023/03/20/best-supplements-to-add-to-your-daily-wellness-routine/

Lestta. (n.d.). *7 tips to improve your digestive health naturally.* Retrieved from https://lestta.com/7-tips-to-improve-your-digestive-health-naturally/

Dr. Efrat LaMandre. (n.d.). *Is your gut health the key to mental wellness?.* Retrieved from https://drefratlamandre.com/is-your-gut-health-the-key-to-mental-wellness/

Discount Supplements Hub. (n.d.). *Healthy Origins Probiotic 30 Billion CFU's.* Retrieved from https://discountsupplementshub.co.uk/product/healthy-origins-probiotic-30-billion-cfus-30-billion-cfu-150-vcaps/

Xanax-Alprazolam. (n.d.). *The connection between probiotics and mental health.* Retrieved from https://xanax-alprazolam.su/the-connection-between-probiotics-and-mental-health

Dubbhism. (n.d.). *How does the microbiota-gut-brain axis influence mental health?.* Retrieved from https://dubbhism.com/archives/658

Frankfurt Bakery. (n.d.). *Foods that boost your vitality.* Retrieved from https://www.frankfurtbakery.com/foods-that-boost-your-vitality/

Align Health Coaching. (2024). *How stress plays a role in your health.* Retrieved from https://alignhealthcoaching.com/2024/01/05/how-stress-plays-a-role-in-your-health/

Coinbit.fi. (n.d.). *The benefits of regular exercise: Enhancing physical and mental well-*

REFERENCES • 189

being. Retrieved from https://coinbit.fi/the-benefits-of-regular-exercise-enhancing-physical-and-mental-well-being/

TYH Wellness. (n.d.). *Get gut happy!!*. Retrieved from https://www.transformingyourhealth.com/blog/get-gut-happy

Moments of Positivity. (n.d.). *Give yourself a boost after a stressful time at work*. Retrieved from https://www.momentsofpositivity.com/web-stories/give-yourself-a-boost

Tranquilia Beds. (n.d.). *Sleep & nutrition: The symbiotic relationship for better health*. Retrieved from https://tranquiliabeds.com.au/blogs/news/sleep-nutrition-the-symbiotic-relationship-for-better-health

White Leaf Nutrition. (n.d.). *The gut feeling: Unleashing the power of prebiotic and probiotic*. Retrieved from https://whiteleafnutritionde.myshopify.com/blogs/news/the-gut-feeling-unleashing-the-power-of-prebiotic-and-probiotic-supplements?shpxid=6448f99c-f36e-4eac-8b8a-060a1816b784

AI Translations. (n.d.). *What are the key differences between a healthy and unhealthy gut microbiome, and how can a person promote a balanced gut flora for overall well-being?*. Retrieved from https://aitranslations.io/knowledge/what_are_the_key_differences_between_a_healthy_and_unhealthy_gut_microbiome_and_how_can_a_person_promote_a_balanced_gut_flora_for_overall_well-being.php

Dr. Naveen Bhadauria. (n.d.). *Is it possible to cure RA permanently?*. Retrieved from https://privatelondonrheumatologist.com/is-it-possible-to-cure-ra-permanently/

DSM East South Chamber. (n.d.). *Anti-inflammatory properties of omega-3*. Retrieved from http://www.dsmeastsouthchamber.org/properties-of-omega-3/

Luma by Laura. (n.d.). *Top herbs for blood sugar*. Retrieved from https://lumabylaura.com/blogs/news/herbs-for-blood-sugar

G-2-C-2. (n.d.). *Shallaki: A natural herbal medicine with anti-inflammatory and anti-arthritic properties*. Retrieved from https://g-2-c-2.org/shallaki-a-natural-herbal-medicine-with-anti-inflammatory-and-anti-arthritic-properties.html

Anxiety Cures Site. (n.d.). *Natural anxiety supplements*. Retrieved from https://anxietycures-site.com/natural-anxiety-supplements/

Innovo US. (n.d.). *Bloating & pelvic floor health link*. Retrieved from https://www.myinnovo.com/blogs/innovo/relationship-between-bloating-and-pelvic-floor-health

Lean Greens. (n.d.). *Natural approaches for gut healing: Restore and optimize your gut health*. Retrieved from https://leangreens.com/blogs/taste/natural-gut-health

TrueHope. (n.d.). *Probiotics and prebiotics for mental health: A guide for families*. Retrieved from https://blog.truehope.com/probiotics-and-prebiotics-for-mental-health-a-guide-for-families/

190 • REFERENCES

Article.pk. (n.d.). *Unlocking microbial marvels: A journey into research.* Retrieved from https://article.pk/researching-the-microbial-marvel-1458

Jonathan Bailor. (n.d.). *Gut health.* Retrieved from https://jonathanbailor.com/gut-health/

TheMindfulMan. (n.d.). *Sensate: Your guide to deep relaxation and better health.* Retrieved from https://themindfulman.io/sensate-your-guide-to-deep-relaxation-and-better-health/

Dr. Maya. (n.d.). *Serotonin and your digestion: The gut-brain connection.* Retrieved from https://doctormayaclinic.com/serotonin_digestion/

Grassland Beef. (n.d.). *What is leaky gut... (And is it the cause of your nagging symptoms?).* Retrieved from https://discover.grasslandbeef.com/blog/what-is-leaky-gut/

Santosh Yoga Institute. (n.d.). *Fasting for mental clarity: Enhance your brain function.* Retrieved from https://santoshyogainstitute.com/fasting-for-mental-clarity/

Hopley, K. (n.d.). *Revitalise your gut health: Insights from gut analysis testing.* Retrieved from https://incorporatingwellnesswithkellyhopley.com/revitalise-your-gut-health-insights-from-gut-analysis-testing/

Sincere Nutrition. (n.d.). *5 signs of an unhealthy gut | Eliminate gases, bloating & indigestion.* Retrieved from https://sincerenutrition.com/blog-signs-of-unhealthy-gut

HugeCount. (n.d.). *12 mindful approaches to eating well.* Retrieved from https://hugecount.com/health/12-mindful-approaches-to-eating-well/

Donna J Wellness. (n.d.). *Intermittent fasting lifestyle.* Retrieved from https://www.donnajwellness.com/blog/tags/intermittent-fasting-lifestyle

Primal Survivor. (n.d.). *Activated charcoal for stomach bugs and diarrhea: Dosage, instructions, and advice.* Retrieved from https://www.primalsurvivor.net/activated-charcoal-stomach-bug/

Health Digest. (n.d.). *When you stop exercising in your 50s, this is what happens to your future health.* Retrieved from https://www.healthdigest.com/1623599/what-happens-to-future-health-stop-exercising-in-50s/

Pakipolitics. (n.d.). *Most the valuable stunning benefits of lemons.* Retrieved from https://pakipolitics.com/most-the-valuable-stunning-benefits-of-lemons/

The Water Cooler Guys. (n.d.). *The morning ritual: Should you drink water as soon as you wake up?.* Retrieved from https://www.thewatercoolerguys.com.au/post/the-morning-ritual-should-you-drink-water-as-soon-as-you-wake-up

Global Care Initiative. (n.d.). *How plant-based diets influence intuitive abilities.* Retrieved from http://www.globalcare-initiative.com/how-plant-based-diets-influence-intuitive-abilities

ProbioticsEverything. (n.d.). *From bloating to bliss: How probiotics can conquer digestive discomfort*. Retrieved from https://probioticseverything.com/from-bloating-to-bliss-how-probiotics-can-conquer-digestive-discomfort/

JustALittleBite. (n.d.). *The mind-body connection: Unraveling the wonders of exercise on mental health*. Retrieved from https://justalittlebite.com/the-mind-body-connection-unraveling-the-wonders-of-exercise-on-mental-health/

GP Acupuncture Oxford. (n.d.). *Irritable bowel syndrome*. Retrieved from https://www.gpacupunctureoxford.co.uk/blog/irritable-bowel-syndrome

Ahead Daily. (n.d.). *7 simple steps to holistic stress relief: The ultimate integration of aromatherapy and other practices*. Retrieved from https://aheaddaily.com/health-medicine/7-simple-steps-to-holistic-stress-relief-the-ultimate-integration-of-aromatherapy-and-other-practices

World Tranquil. (n.d.). *Aromatherapy*. Retrieved from https://worldtranquil.com/aromatherapy/

MeArticles. (n.d.). *The secret to boosting gut microbiome diversity for optimal health*. Retrieved from https://www.mearticles.com/2023/07/the-secret-to-boosting-gut-microbiome.html

ARTAH. (n.d.). *What really happens when we don't eat enough fibre*. Retrieved from https://artah.co/blogs/journal/what-really-happens-when-we-dont-eat-enough-fibre

Carolina Pain Scrambler Center. (2020). *Lifestyle for people with chronic pain*. Retrieved from https://carolinapainscrambler.com/2020/01/13/lifestyle-for-people-with-chronic-pain/

Dodhisattva. (n.d.). *How to increase GABA: 5 effective ways to increase GABA for mental health and anxiety relief*. Retrieved from https://dodhisattva.com/how-to-increase-gaba/

PureHealth Research. (n.d.). *How to fix your leaky gut: 8 tips*. Retrieved from https://blog.purehealthresearch.com/how-to-fix-a-leaky-gut/

Healthy Guts. (n.d.). *Gut health diet 101: Your ultimate guide to digestive bliss*. Retrieved from https://healthyguts.net/gut-health-diet-101-your-ultimate-guide-to-digestive-bliss/

New Eden School of Natural Health. (n.d.). *10 natural hacks to improve gut health*. Retrieved from https://www.newedenschoolofnaturalhealth.org/gut-health/

Total Balanced Health. (n.d.). *Dandelions: Can't beat them? Eat them!*. Retrieved from https://totalbalancedhealth.com/dandelions-cant-beat-them-eat-them/

Oter.app. (n.d.). *Cultivate a growth mindset from "summary" of The Power of a Positive Team by Jon Gordon*. Retrieved from https://oter.app/posts/the-power-of-a-positive-team-cultivate-a-growth-mindset-1?source=similar-post

Lose Weight Fastx. (n.d.). *Healthy habit formation*. Retrieved from https://lose-weight-fastx.com/healthy-habit-formation/

Mindbody and Soul. (n.d.). *Definition and importance of discipline in personal growth*.

192 • REFERENCES

Retrieved from https://mindbody-and-soul.com/definition-and-importance-of-discipline-in-personal-growth/

Greenlife Wellness. (n.d.). *Health and wellness education*. Retrieved from https://greenlifewellness.co.ke/services/health-and-wellness-education/

Gut Pathogens. (n.d.). *Gut pathogens and mental health*. Retrieved from https://gutpathogens.biomedcentral.com/articles/10.1186/s13099-020-0346-1?utm_source=chatgpt.com

Frontiers in Cellular and Infection Microbiology. (2022). *Stress and the gut-brain axis: Mechanisms and implications*. Retrieved from https://www.frontiersin.org/journals/cellular-and-infection-microbiology/articles/10.3389/fcimb.2022.915701/full?utm_source=chatgpt.com

MDPI. (2023). *The gut-brain connection and its impact on health*. Retrieved from https://www.mdpi.com/1422-0067/24/23/16660?utm_source=chatgpt.com

Journal of Pharmaceutical Health Care and Sciences. (2019). *Gut microbiota and its role in stress-related disorders*. Retrieved from https://jphcs.biomedcentral.com/articles/10.1186/s40780-019-0148-0?utm_source=chatgpt.com

WCHSB Insights. (2024). *Stress relief with acupuncture and aromatherapy*. Retrieved from https://insights.wchsb.com/2024/07/03/stress-relief-with-acupuncture-and-aromatherapy/?utm_source=chatgpt.com

Santos, J., et al. (2021). Stress and the gut-brain axis: Implications for health. *Neurobiology of Stress*.

Kelly, J. R., et al. (2015). Stress and the gut microbiota: Mechanisms and effects on health. *Frontiers in Microbiology*.

Knowles, S. R., et al. (2018). The gut-brain axis and its role in stress-related disorders. *Brain, Behavior, and Immunity*.

Benson, S., et al. (2019). Cortisol and its effects on gastrointestinal symptoms. *Psychoneuroendocrinology*.

Knowles, S. R., et al. (2018). Chronic stress, gut dysbiosis, and microbiota-related diseases. *Brain, Behavior, and Immunity*.

O'Mahony, S. M., et al. (2020). The impact of stress on gut permeability and inflammation. *Nutrients*.

Heijnen, S., et al. (2019). Exercise, stress, and cortisol: Their role in gut health. *The Journal of Sports Science & Medicine*.

Creswell, J. D., et al. (2021). Mindfulness techniques for stress reduction and cortisol control. *Psychosomatic Medicine*.

Perciavalle, V., et al. (2017). The role of deep breathing on stress reduction. *Psychosomatic Medicine*.

Creswell, J. D., et al. (2014). Mindfulness-based stress reduction improves sleep and reduces anxiety. *JAMA Internal Medicine*.

Creswell, J. D., et al. (2016). Mindfulness meditation reduces cortisol and stress responses. *Biological Psychiatry.*

Knowles, S. R., et al. (2018). The gut-brain axis and mindfulness interventions. *Brain, Behavior, and Immunity.*

Printed in Great Britain
by Amazon